Quality of Life in Asia

Volume 20

This series, the first of its kind, examines both the objective and subjective dimensions of life quality in Asia, especially East Asia. It unravels and compares the contours, dynamics and patterns of building nations by offering innovative works that discuss basic and applied research and emphasizing inter- and multi-disciplinary approaches to the various domains of life quality. The series appeals to a variety of fields in humanities, social sciences and other professional disciplines. Asia is the largest, most populous continent on Earth, and it is home to the world's most dynamic region, East Asia. In the past three decades, East Asia has been the most successful region in the world in expanding its economies and integrating them into the global economy, offering lessons on how poor countries, even with limited natural resources, can achieve rapid economic development. Yet while scholars and policymakers have focused on why East Asia has prospered, little has been written on how its economic expansion has affected the quality of life of its citizens. This series publish several volumes a year, either single or multiple-authored monographs or collections of essays.

Cahyo Pamungkas · Gusti Ayu Ketut Surtiari ·
Sari Seftiani
Editors

The Impact of the Pandemic on Indigenous People in Indonesia

Socio-Demographic Perspectives after COVID-19

BRIN
BADAN RISET
DAN INOVASI NASIONAL

Springer

Editors
Cahyo Pamungkas
Research Center for Area Studies
National Research and Innovation Agency (BRIN)
Jakarta, Indonesia

Gusti Ayu Ketut Surtiari
Research Center for Population
National Research and Innovation Agency (BRIN)
Jakarta, Indonesia

Sari Seftiani
Research Center for Population
National Research and Innovation Agency (BRIN)
Jakarta, Indonesia

ISSN 2211-0550 ISSN 2211-0569 (electronic)
Quality of Life in Asia
ISBN 978-981-96-4221-2 ISBN 978-981-96-4222-9 (eBook)
https://doi.org/10.1007/978-981-96-4222-9

Jointly published with BRIN Publishing

This Springer imprint is published by the registered company Springer Nature Singapore Pte Ltd.
The registered company address is: 152 Beach Road, #21-01/04 Gateway East, Singapore 189721, Singapore

Foreword

This book on the impact of COVID-19 on Indigenous People in Indonesia recounts the following incident:

> In the midst of COVID-19, Tenggerese villagers in the highlands of East Java were gathering in front of the house of the village head to perform the *tayuban*, a traditional dance ritual held to pray for the ancestors and engender communal harmony. The local COVID-19 Task Force arrived to close down the event, following the government's Regulation to Restrict Community Activities (PPKM). A stand-off ensued: participants in the ritual believed that the spirits of their ancestors were not happy with this unilateral action; some locals were possessed by these spirits, cursing and threatening the Task Force for forcibly shutting down the event. The Task Force backed off and the event resumed and concluded.

This event demonstrates the main argument of the book: COVID-19 was not just a contagious viral disease, to be treated through medical procedures and preventative public health measures; for governments and health professionals charged with minimizing mortality, illness and contagion, treating COVID-19 required understanding of the socio-cultural contexts in which it was playing out; and for researchers studying the impacts of COVID-19 afterwards, it is imperative to understand the differing perceptions of COVID-19 and the socioeconomic conditions and worldviews among different groups. In many contexts in Indonesia, as this book shows, the Indigenous People were not fazed by COVID-19: they discounted its severity, relied upon their tried-and-true herbal remedies for coughs and colds and 'flu, sometimes withdrew to homelands and restricted mobility, and in many cases, as above, continued to perform their traditional community rituals which, they believed, warded off malevolent forces and gave them immunity to externally generated diseases.

At the outset of COVID-19, globally, and in many countries such as Australia (Commonwealth of Australia 2024), Indigenous People were identified as being particularly vulnerable because of their historical and structural disadvantage: they are often located far from health, education and WASH (water, sanitation and hygiene) facilities; they often experience pre-existing poverty, low levels of education, poor health and premature mortality; they are often situated at the margins of mainstream society and the worldwide market economy, and suffer stigmatization; they are sometimes barely touched by government and modern media. This picture of uniform Indigenous vulnerability to COVID-19 is tested in this book.

First, in Indonesia, "there is no single definition that can classify all [the] indigenous peoples." The absence of a national formal definition, and of criteria for establishing indigeneity, has meant that the national Bureau of Statistics does not collect statistics on "Indigenous People" in Indonesia. Establishing the mortality rates and demographic impacts of COVID-19 on Indigenous People in Indonesia is therefore well-nigh impossible, though this book makes some attempts to quantify mortality, fertility and migration impacts of COVID-19 in its case study areas. Age group and gender were identified as showing patterns. While some statistics in this book show that the rate of exposure to COVID-19 and the concomitant COVID-19 mortality rate of Indigenous People was high among those of productive ages, rather than among the elderly, it should also be noted that among some Indigenous groups, there are very few people aged over 60 years (e.g., Sudibyo and Parker 2024: 204), and 60 years is the cut-off for "the elderly" age-group in Indonesian statistics. What does seem clear is that gender made a difference: while women had high rates of exposure, it was mostly the men who died made vulnerable by high rates of smoking.

Indigenous groups in Indonesia are diverse: they live in every kind of settlement ranging from cities to villages to nomadic family units; some are isolated forest-dwellers, some live in sedentary villages, others are well integrated into the urban, educated middle classes; some practice their own belief systems and others follow one of the Great Religious Traditions. In this book, seven groups were investigated by the all-Indonesian group of researchers: from west to east, the Orang Rimba in Jambi, Sumatra, the Tenggerese in mountainous East Java, the Bali Aga in Bali, the Marapu in Sumba, East Nusa Tenggara, the Tugutil in Halmahera, North Maluku, the Nuaulu in Seram, Maluku and the Orang Asli Papua in Biak, Papua.

The great strength of this edited collection is its understanding that among different Indigenous groups, perceptions of COVID-19 varied. Perceptions were shaped by people's knowledge, prior experiences, worldviews and religious beliefs, degree of physical remoteness and integration with larger economic, knowledge and political systems, and emotions such as fear and (mis)trust. The other great strength is the concomitant of the first: this variety of perceptions, socio-economic and even political contexts, meant that the social and demographic impacts of COVID-19 were diverse.

Some Indigenous People, such as the Tenggerese and the Bali Aga, are well integrated into the international tourist economy. When the tourist economy collapsed, they retreated to their home villages, attempting to revert to agricultural livelihoods. Economic impacts were severe: among these groups, incomes dropped and unemployment rose. But the incident with which this Foreword began shows that this economic integration into the global, late capitalist economy did not stop them relying on traditional beliefs about the need to keep the ancestors happy. Others, such as the Orang Rimba and the Tugutil, are mostly nomadic peoples living deep in the jungle. These groups sometimes pulled back, restricting their mobility and market interactions with town-dwellers, relying upon their traditional herbs and rituals to keep them immune, but underestimated the contagion potential of COVID-19 among themselves. Some drops in income were evident as a result of a decline in trading; some groups adapted by restricting the range of food items consumed, and the number of meals per day.

Beliefs about the causes of COVID-19 were varied. The Nuaulu, for instance, believe there is a close relationship between sins and the outbreak of disease. According to a local community leader, "The Almighty knows that those who make the greatest mistakes will suffer the most diseases." The Usi Rosa is a traditional procession that aims to atone for sins. In October 2020, more than a hundred Nuaulu adults performed the Usi Rosa to prevent the spread of COVID-19 in their region. Such congregations were seen as super-spreader events by medical authorities and banned by government. The performance can be seen as evidence of the ineffectiveness of government messaging and its inability to bridge the gap between biomedical science and traditional worldviews.

In mainstream Indonesia, Papuans are often disparaged as primitive savages. But in the Papua case study, those who live in urban areas are employed in the government bureaucracy, as teachers, medical personnel and priests, and in markets as sellers of areca nut, woven bags and agricultural products; islanders are typically cultivators, copra producers, and fishers. Some Papuans had a group memory of the disastrous Spanish flu epidemic of a century earlier and of the depredations of cholera and STIs. For the Papuans, the political context was also influential: many feared and mistrusted the government, against the backdrop of the Papuan independence movement and Jakarta's often violent attempt to quell it, and the massive inflow of transmigrants from elsewhere in Indonesia, making them a minority in their own land. Mis- and dis-information about the spread of COVID-19 on social media was rife, and many believed that it was being spread to wipe out the Indigenous Papuans (*dikovidkan*). One notable act of resistance was a boatload of escapees, disobeying the government lockdown in Numfor Island: the authorities burned the boat to punish the escapees and show their serious intent.

Papuans displayed ambivalence about COVID-19. Many Papuans, especially those in rural areas, denied the presence of it, and yet believed that testing positive for COVID-19 was a disgrace to their extended family. One woman who tested positive asked the clinic to keep her disease a secret: they agreed, she was instructed to self-isolate and wear a face mask, but was later seen by researchers walking around her village as usual. One tribal chief believed it was God's curse on humankind, similar to the Biblical flood sent in Noah's day, due to people's avarice, environmental destruction and the ever-widening gap between the rich and poor. Some saw it as a manifestation of God's wrath and a sign that people must repent their sins. Others saw it in global politico-apocalyptic terms, as a precursor to a great catastrophe: World War III. COVID-19 could only be averted by prayers, repentance, worship and good behaviour, practicing peace and compassion among humans and God's other creatures.

In Bali, the Bali Aga managed a reasonable compromise between their traditional worldview and medical regulations. The Balinese believe in the co-existence and co-dependence of the seen (*sekala*) and unseen (*niskala*) worlds. The village head, the *bendesa*, wore "two hats": he was both the head of the village COVID-19 Task Force, responsible for compliance with the public health measures—the "seen" actions—and the traditional leader, responsible for the performance of rituals and processions to ward off misfortune wrought by COVID-19 (the "unseen"). The rituals were performed ten times during COVID-19, but participation was limited to 15 persons.

COVID-19 tested leaders at every level around the world—from the Director of the World Health Organisation (WHO), to national leaders, down to the neighborhood level.

Leadership involved balancing the "public good," the resilience of the state health system and especially the vulnerability of minorities, with individual rights to freedom of movement and livelihoods. Among the Indigenous Peoples of Indonesia, this was complicated by their common perception that COVID-19 was not a significant threat to their life, and that their traditional ways could be relied upon to help them overcome such challenge as it posed. This study found that in the research sites, Indigenous People relied heavily on their customary leaders for guidance and orders, and that obedience to Indigenous leaders was the most important factor in responding to the crisis.

Testing and tracing were not well implemented in Indonesia. Although mask-wearing regulations were not notably successful away from public buildings such as government offices, Indigenous People mostly complied with other directives from government authority figures, such as the prohibition of movement from area to area. However, government regulations were not always consistent, with spikes of massive population movement around Eid Al-fitr (*Idulfitri*), for example. Distrust of the vaccines and of hospitals—places where people go to die—and the persistence of the performance of "super-spreader" traditional rituals, processions and dances show that COVID-19 often exacerbated the gap between traditional Indigenous worldviews of health and disease on the one hand and the biomedical model of health care and illness prevention on the other.

It is five years since the WHO pronounced COVID-19 a global pandemic (March 11, 2020). While we lack good statistics for the incidence and mortality rate of COVID-19 in Indonesia, we can now step back and see some patterns and learnings. I commend this book to you as a timely and useful collection of essays that points the way for preparation for the next global health crisis. It shows that we need to improve the health and science education of all people in Indonesia; that medical and government personnel need to develop inclusiveness in accommodating the life-worlds of Indigenous People, to be mindful of the different priorities and sometimes clashing epistemologies of culture and medicine, and to take the time to work out compromises that will keep people safe and well; that Indigenous People were right to withdraw from interaction with others, but that this needed to be followed up with effective vaccination distribution and education. It is important that Indonesia develop a balanced, proportionate, and adaptable response to the next global health crisis, a response that minimizes death and illness, protects the health system, and minimizes the widening of existing health, social, and economic inequities.

Lyn Parker
School of Social Sciences
The University of Western Australia
Perth, Australia

References

Commonwealth of Australia, Department of the Prime Minister and Cabinet, 2024, COVID-19 Response Inquiry Report. Available at https://www.pmc.gov.au/resources/COVID-19-response-inquiry-report.

Sudibyo, L., & Lyn P. (2024):.'Menjadi Manusia' (Becoming Somebody): The Aspirations and Realities of Marind Young People, Papua, Indonesia, Ocenia, *94*(3), 202–223. https://doi.org/10.1002/ocea.5417.

Contents

Chapter 1
Introduction: Indigenous People in the Struggle Against COVID-19

Intan Adhi Perdana Putri, Nailatalmuna Nitrasatri Atmaja, and Sari Seftiani

Abstract This chapter contains the background that explains why the COVID-19 pandemic should be seen beyond the health problems. In this chapter, Putri et al. reveal the importance of gaining better understanding about the COVID-19 pandemic through a sociodemographic perspective and illustrate the reasons why the indigenous people are considered to be a vulnerable group that is at higher risk of exposure to the pandemic. However, we also question whether indigenous peoples are the most vulnerable groups or resilient in facing the COVID-19 pandemic. The second subtitle describes the impacts of the COVID-19 pandemic on indigenous people from previous studies, especially related to demographics such as mobility patterns, fertility rates, mortality rates, and livelihood. Besides the vulnerabilities and impacts of the COVID-19 pandemic that are understood from sociodemographic perspectives, this chapter also represents how indigenous peoples perceive, respond, and adapt to the COVID-19 pandemic. In addition, Putri et al. explain the data source and locus of indigenous people where we researched and provide detailed information regarding indigenous people who are learned in our research.

Keywords Indigenous people · COVID-19 · Pandemic · Sociodemographic perspective

The pandemic of coronavirus disease 2019 (COVID-19), which in Indonesia began in March 2020, has shook and disturbed human life and posed unprecedented challenges to the world's health, systems, and working realm (Chriscaden, 2020). According to the World Health Organization (WHO, 2020), this virus attacks the respiratory system and spreads rapidly. By the end of January 2022, this virus caused 7.01

I. A. P. Putri (✉) · S. Seftiani
Research Center for Population, National Research and Innovation Agency (BRIN), Jakarta, Indonesia
e-mail: intan.adhi.perdana.putri@brin.go.id

N. N. Atmaja
Directorate for Economy, Employment, and Regional Development Policy, National Research and Innovation Agency (BRIN), Jakarta, Indonesia

C. Pamungkas et al. (eds.), *The Impact of the Pandemic on Indigenous People in Indonesia*, Quality of Life in Asia 20, https://doi.org/10.1007/978-981-96-4222-9_1

million deaths (Wordometer, 2024). The systemic effects of the pandemic have been shown also across all sectors of society in many countries, including Indonesia. More than 144,000 Indonesian individuals have died from this virus as of January 31, 2023 (Satuan Tugas Penanganan COVID-19, 2020), while 21.32 million people of working age were impacted by layoffs, temporary unemployment, or reduced hours (BPS, 2021a). In addition, the tourism industry was suffering due to the lockdown policy. Besides its effects on the economy, the COVID-19 pandemic has influenced sociodemographic factors such as births, deaths, and migration (Ullah et al., 2020).

Various stakeholders have been concerned about how the COVID-19 pandemic would affect vulnerable communities in particular. Indigenous people are among those considered to be at higher risk of exposure to the pandemic. Anne Nourgam, Chairperson of United Nations Permanent Forum on Indigenous Issues, said that indigenous peoples' vulnerabilities were due to their pre-existing limited access to healthcare even prior to the outbreak of the pandemic. They may face a higher rate of infection because of, among other things, poor access to essential services like sanitation, education, and housing, as well as difficulties to obtain transmission preventive measures like soap, masks, and disinfectants (United Nations, 2020). According to Nourgam (2020), many of indigenous people might have been living in extreme poverty, malnourishment, and inadequate immunity, therefore leaving them even more susceptible to the infectious disease.

Indigenous peoples, despite their disadvantages, play a unique and crucial role in the preservation of land and ecosystems. The fact that their areas are home to 80% of the world's biodiversity is inseparable from the local knowledge they have acquired thus far (IFAD, 2020). More than 476 million indigenous peoples (about 6.2% of the world's population) are dispersed throughout 90 nations and live in both urban and rural settings (United Nation, 2020). AMAN (The Indigenous Peoples' Alliance of the Archipelago) reports that in Indonesia there are 70 million indigenous peoples and 2371 of them are enrolled members of the independent civil organization (Andiarsi, 2020).

Indonesia's indigenous peoples, with their wide range of social and cultural traditions, may be found all over the country's islands. It is not uncommon for them to reside in cities, villages, or even the forest, with a variety of livelihoods ranging from plantations and agriculture to tourism and academia with some even making it to the high levels of political office. In addition, there are still nomadic and semi-nomadic indigenous peoples in Indonesia who rely on hunting and gathering as their primary source of income. Given this variation, the responses provided and the effects felt by Indonesia's indigenous people in reaction to the COVID-19 pandemic are undoubtedly diverse and, therefore, must be documented in a book. This volume will explore the situation of several indigenous peoples during the pandemic as well as their adaptation strategies.

1.1 Indigenous Peoples: The Most Vulnerable or Resilient?

Recent studies on vulnerability, particularly in light of the COVID-19 pandemic, have heavily embraced Fineman's vulnerability theory (2017) (Denny et al., 2021; Fitzmaurice, 2021; Gordon-Bouvier, 2021; Kiwnuka, 2021; Jobe, 2021; Siriwardhane & Khan, 2021). Fineman (2018) claimed that her concept of vulnerability is designed specifically to make the state more responsive and egalitarian. Gordon-Bouvier (2021) argues that Martha Fineman's description of vulnerability is more evident when linked to the COVID-19 pandemic, where common vulnerabilities are becoming increasingly obvious and are compounded by large disparities in people's unequal access to resilience. In addition, no one is born resilient, but with the help of institutions and social ties, resiliency can be developed over time.

Wisner et al. (2004) provide another theory of vulnerability, focusing on natural hazards and the qualities of individuals or groups in specific situations that determine their capacity to anticipate, cope with, and endure the effects of calamities. Hazardous events can have a negative impact on all aspects of the affected peoples, indigenous peoples in this case, including their livelihoods and assets, all of which are examined in terms of disaster vulnerability (Cardona et al., 2012). The two perspectives on vulnerability (either from Fineman or Wisner and other scholars in the field of disaster) are still relevant to the conditions and characteristics of indigenous people's vulnerability that will be discussed in this book, especially those related to the COVID-19 pandemic.

Indigenous peoples have always been seen as a vulnerable group, in part due to their lack of access to mainstream services in healthcare, housing, economy, and others. According to Millalen et al. (2020), indigenous peoples continue to be vulnerable in terms of illness prevention and treatment due to poverty and systemic racism in health policies. In other words, indigenous peoples continue to be treated the same way as the rest of society in terms of fundamental amenities such as education and housing, which remains a concern for diverse stakeholders, particularly those who care about indigenous peoples inhibiting the interior areas. Furthermore, the number of indigenous peoples infected by coronavirus is still not clearly known. According to Araujo et al. (2021), this lack of information is due to the insufficient tracing coverage for indigenous peoples, despite the fact that death and morbidity rates for indigenous peoples in several locations of the world are higher than those of other groups.

According to the available data, the death rate among indigenous peoples in Brazil, for example, is 4.1% higher than the national average (Milhorance, 2021). Another illustration is New Zealand, where the infection mortality rate among the Māoris is half times greater than that of the non-Māoris (Steyn et al., 2020). In contrast to other nations, Indonesia lacks records, documentations, and publications about the number of indigenous people afflicted by and died from this virus. This is so unfortunate given the fact that data is of importance to understand the dynamics and conditions of Indonesia's indigenous communities in relation to the COVID-19 pandemic, as well as to serve as a future reference for dealing with similar situations.

In addition to being vulnerable to the aforementioned factors, indigenous peoples whose livelihoods depend on tourism are also undergoing significant shocks (World Tourism Organization, 2021; Cord & Pizarro, 2021). Therefore, one recommendation suggests that indigenous people should have multiple sources of income so that they are less vulnerable in the future when faced with similar situations. It is true that indigenous peoples are the most vulnerable in the midst of the COVID-19 pandemic, as indicated in several articles and researches. Nourgam (2020), however, contends that indigenous peoples can also help to finding answers in this era of the COVID-19 pandemic, for instance through good practices in traditional knowledge and medicine. As an illustration, many people around the world are now modeling indigenous communities' practice of self-imposed isolation. By banning the entry of various outside movements, indigenous peoples swiftly restrict mobility within their societies based on customary norms (GEF, 2020). Undoubtedly, this is their method of utilizing the knowledge that has been passed down from generation to generation regarding how to prevent the transmission of disease.

Other traditional knowledge is the practice of helping each other and making sure people in need, be it family members, friends or the community, get the support they need; indigenous communities in Peru call this kind of traditional custom Apachicuy which means "help the love ones" (FAO, 2020). In addition to traditional wisdom in preventing the spread of the virus, GEF (2020) identifies additional strengths in the form of a number of traditional treatments that look promising in fighting viruses, including COVID-19. Cord & Pizarro (2021) added that their access to natural resources enables them to produce food through agriculture and plantations.

The question is thus whether indigenous peoples are vulnerable or resilient. The diverse features of indigenous peoples across the world generate diverse factors of vulnerability and resilience. Identifying and documenting the variables behind the vulnerability and resilience of each indigenous people is crucial for determining what can be done to make indigenous peoples more resilient in the face of several disruptions, such as the COVID-19 pandemic. There are a lot of different things that could be considered in mitigating the vulnerability of indigenous peoples, including that their traditional wisdom could be adopted by the society in general.

1.2 The Bad and the Ugly Truth About the Impacts of COVID-19 on Indigenous Peoples

The COVID-19 pandemic has had a number of unpredicted consequences in Indonesia. A survey by BPS-Statistics Indonesia in 2020 showed that the pandemic has resulted in a wide range of societal changes and patterns of adaptation, including those in transportation, employment, education, and disaster-related mental attitudes (BPS, 2020). The high mortality rate of those infected with COVID-19 is the most significant impact. COVID-19 fatalities in Indonesia are among the highest in the world, according to the World Health Organization (Dihni, 2021).

In addition to the high death rate, male infertility has been linked to COVID-19 infection according to a number of studies (Huan et al., 2021; Vishvkarma & Rajender, 2020). The pandemic may also lead to a baby boom. During the period of Large-Scale Social Restrictions (PSBB) most people are staying at home, which will likely affect the fertility rates because of increased sexual intercourse between husband and wife and decreased access to contraception since individuals are not permitted to leave the house. According to National Population and Family Planning Board (BKKBN) statistics, the usage of contraceptives dropped by 10% between March and April 2020, resulting in an additional 300,000 to 450,000 births assuming 15% of those women subsequently become pregnant (Souisa et al., 2020).

The COVID-19 pandemic has also changed migration patterns. The changing trend in mobility patterns is found in nearly every province of Indonesia as a response to the Work from Home and PSBB policy (BPS, 2020). In addition, this shift in movement patterns has had a significant influence on the community's economic and social aspects. Geoffrey Garrett said that the COVID-19 pandemic has slowed down urbanization because individuals are more cautious about their movements while avoiding crowds identical to daily patterns of urban life (Garrett, 2020).

The aforementioned sociodemographic effects can be even worse for indigenous peoples who are frequently excluded from the formal state-provided social protection system, leaving many without access to emergency healthcare and financial assistance. The Economic Commission for Latin America and the Caribbean (ECLAC) (2021) revealed that in Latin America, despite a lower aging in indigenous peoples' population structures, two factors may expose older indigenous individuals to a larger risk of infection and a more severe disease effect than their non-indigenous counterparts. Indigenous peoples have a longer working period, during which older members continue to play an active part, but their status as informal laborers limit their access to the social security system. Consequently, the pandemic has a bigger effect on the death rate among indigenous populations. Millalen et al. (2020) concluded that a greater proportion of indigenous-populated regions such as those in Chile are not only more vulnerable to the virus, but also have more COVID-19-related mortality. An insufficient healthcare system prior to COVID-19 also contributed to this condition.

Women and children are one of the indigenous peoples' most vulnerable groups. COVID-19 has made indigenous women have less access to sexual and reproductive health services. The medical personnel are preoccupied with combating COVID-19, and thereby forbidding them to provide the services. Furthermore, health clinics in many areas are shutting or restricting their services, which makes it difficult for women to get these treatments. Women also refuse to visit related service facilities out of fear of infection and restricted movement prevents them from gaining access to comprehensive health services. Supply chains are also disrupted too, reducing the availability of drugs, including contraceptive methods (ECLAC, 2021).

Indigenous peoples have strong ties to their communities, the land, and nature. Consequently, their economies have traditionally revolved around tourism, agriculture, mining, and art production (Leach et al., 2020; APEC, 2021). The pandemic affects all sectors that provide the primary means of subsistence for indigenous peoples who therefore cannot access global marketplaces to sell their agricultural, livestock, and handicraft products (IWGIA, 2021; APEC, 2021). Markets are closed, and transportation is unavailable, as a result of stringent lockdown measures. Indigenous people' inability to sell their goods in local markets contributes directly to the loss of their sources of income. A decline or absence of tourists has a devastating impact on hospitality and tourism industries, resulting in an enormous loss of income for indigenous peoples such as those in Canada and Australia (ILO, 2020; APEC, 2021). Due to the drop in tourism caused by the pandemic, indigenous peoples no longer have jobs, sources of money, or the means to purchase food. In addition, the constraints that hinder indigenous peoples from entering the formal labor force prevent them from having access to social safety nets, thus they do not have a regular income during the pandemic.

Sociodemographic aspects, particularly when they come to indigenous peoples, must be taken into account and used as a foundation for grasping the current situation. In general, all demographic elements are necessary not only to respond to the varied implications of the socio-health crisis on indigenous peoples, but also to pay attention to the possible impacts of prevention, containment, and mitigation efforts. By comprehending these demographic facets, the pandemic case curve can be actually drawn, facilitating policy formulation, particularly for the state, in regards to indigenous populations.

1.3 Responses and Adaptation Strategies

The COVID-19 pandemic has had a significant influence on the life of indigenous peoples. While indigenous peoples have inherent vulnerabilities, it is essential to understand features that distinguish how they perceive, respond, and adapt to the COVID-19 pandemic. The extent to which indigenous peoples perceive the COVID-19 pandemic determines responses and adaptation strategies being taken. Due to the limitations that indigenous peoples have, their responses and solutions are frequently facing numerous challenges.

It is essential to observe and understand how indigenous peoples have responded to the COVID-19 pandemic in the wake of the restrictions and marginalization-related difficulties they have encountered thus far. In addition, it is intriguing to learn about indigenous peoples' local knowledge of COVID-19, since it provides lessons for managing COVID-19 in Indonesia. By understanding the specificity of impacts on indigenous peoples and combining infection curve models from epidemiology with social network models, demographers have been able to create simulations demonstrating how different types of social network interactions between similar people residing in close-knit communities can aid in the gradual reduction of territorial quarantine measures or lockdowns (Block et al., 2020).

Responses to indigenous peoples are not limited to the level of the individuals or the community. It is also important to consider how the government responds to the pandemic on behalf of its marginalized population, the indigenous peoples.

Araujo et al. (2021) offer suggestions for what the government should do, particularly in providing short- and long-term remedies to the pandemic in relation to indigenous communities. The short-term responses include (1) promoting indigenous-led initiatives; (2) collaborating with shamans and other indigenous specialists; (3) involving indigenous women's organizations; (4) working with indigenous youth; (5) respecting indigenous peoples; (6) developing information strategies; (7) facilitating emergency access to water, sanitation, and hygiene (WASH); (8) putting in place emergency referral services and mechanisms, such as field treatment centers; (9) giving indigenous peoples access to their agricultural land; and (10) ensuring emergency cash transfers.

For the Totonac people of Mexico, health and food systems are inextricably linked, and plantations provide them sustenance and therapeutic herbs they are using for immunity-building purposes during the pandemic (APEC, 2021). Walters et al. (2021) mentioned that the Mayan indigenous peoples of Guatemala develop therapies using ginger, garlic, eucalyptus, and honey, occasionally combined with conventional medicine, to boost their immunological response. After locating and cultivating indigenous plants in their ancestral lands, indigenous peoples plant them in their backyards in a communal protected system. Indigenous peoples with access to natural resources are able to farm, collect, and mobilize finances to address the community's urgent needs prior to receiving external aid. When the Chilean Government put an end to its lockdown policy in their territories, the Rapa Nui peoples on Easter Island of Chile implemented a mass quarantine in order to control the infection. They declared themselves to be in Tapu (a state of self-care and community protection) and kept the area off-limits to outsiders.

According to Araujo et al. (2021), the government can implement the following long-term adaptation strategies so that indigenous peoples can recover: (1) proactively (re)building trust; (2) highlighting the key significance of indigenous communal care; (3) improving financing for indigenous health services and addressing health inequities; (4) working with shamanic practitioners and other indigenous experts; (5) investing in WASH on a larger scale; and (6) scaling up social protection; and (7) providing stable internet access.

1.4 Data Sources and Locus of Indigenous Peoples in the Book

This book focuses on the vulnerability of Indonesia's indigenous peoples to the pandemic and its impacts on sociodemographic trends as well as their response and adaptation measures. The communities shown in this book do not yet reflect all indigenous peoples in Indonesia. Nonetheless, this book at least attempts to provide a picture of several indigenous peoples in their responses to the COVID-19 pandemic. The indigenous peoples captured in this book reveals a geographic distribution of Jambi (Orang Rimba), East Java (Tengger), Bali (Bali Aga), East Nusa Tenggara

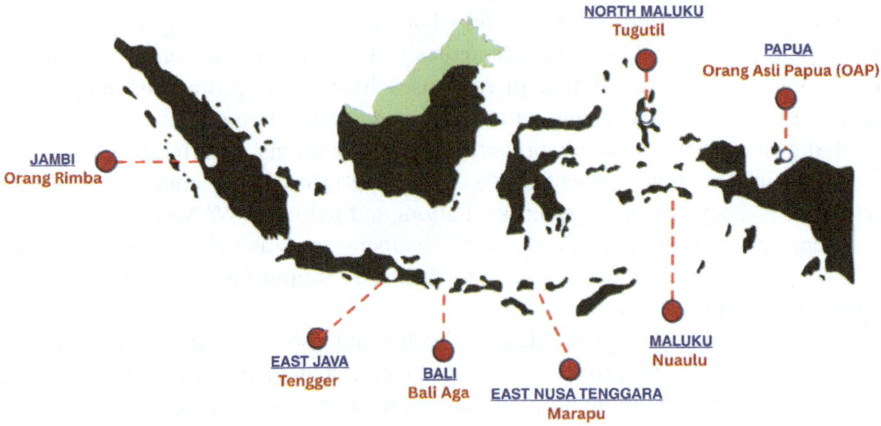

Fig. 1.1 Research sites of indigenous peoples

(NTT) (Marapu), Maluku (Nuaulu), North Maluku (Tugutil), and Papua (Orang Asli Papua).

The following figure shows the research sites of the indigenous peoples in further detail (Fig. 1.1).

1. Orang Rimba

   Orang Rimba literally means "People of the Jungle." In general, the Orang Rimba make a living from hunting and gathering, referred to in some literature as economic hunter-gatherers who rely on exchanges of natural resources for economic activities (Prasetijo, 2017). The Orang Rimba is basically a nomadic tribe who are moving from place to place according to the cycles and the courses of their land-openings. The Orang Rimba referred to in this book are the Orang Rimba of Jambi Province living in the Bukit Dua Belas National Park, the Orang Rimba inhabiting oil palm farms, and the Orang Rimba staying or being relocated in resettlements.

2. Tengger

   The Tengger people are living around the Semeru areas with strong customs and traditions like Karo and Kasada, as well as rites like Sayut for pregnancy, Among-among for birth, and Entas-entas for death. Ngadas Village is one of the Tengger's native enclaves that still survive. The Tengger in Ngadas believe that Tengger is not an identity, but rather a philosophy of life enshrined in ritual ceremonies being performed throughout one's life cycle. More than ninety percent of the Tengger population in Ngadas Village depend on agriculture as their chief means of livelihoods. Another additional source of income is tourism: the average Tengger are jeep owners, jeep rental operators, homestay hosts, small shopkeepers (meatballs, coffee, t-shirts, etc.), and brokers (*keber*).

3. Bali Aga or Bali Mula

   The research in Bali focused on the indigenous people of Bali known as the Bali Aga or others might call it the Bali Mula. However, the fieldwork found that there are two characteristics of the Bali Aga. The first refers to the Bali Aga living in the areas of Catur Desa Dalem Adat Tamblingan that consists of four villages, i.e., Umajero Village, Gobleg Village, Munduk Village, and Gesing Village. The second belongs to the Bali Aga in five villages that have just been inaugurated as the Bali Aga villages or the Mahagotra Panca Desa Bali Aga known as SCTPB, i.e., Sidatapa Village, Cempaga Village, Tigawasa Village, Pedawa Village, and Banyusri Village. In general, the difference between the two groups of Bali Aga is relatively small. The People of Bali Aga in the Dalem Adat Tamblingan are those individuals who have inhibited Bali since the early history of the area and believe that they belong to the religion of Piagem Game Tirta or uphold the nobility of water sources in the Tamblingan Lake area. As for those living in the Mahagotra Panca Desa Bali Aga, they are classified as members of the Bali Aga because the local communities believe so. They could also include migrants from other places in Bali provided that they have fully carried out the traditions and all mutual agreements in the village.

   In general, the people of Bali Aga were those who lived in the villages situated at the Bali's highlands and were less influenced by the Majapahit invasion in 1343 (Reuter, 2005; Pitana, 1994). Their culture is distinct from that of the Majapahit Bali (mainland Bali). The contrasts include that the "The People of Bali Aga" adopt a religious practice in which the dead is not cremated; they do not recognize a caste system in social life; they do not consult with the Brahmin priests (*pedanda*); and they do not read sacred chants (*mantras*) in Sanskrit when praying. Geographically, the five villages, all of which are located in dry areas, have a high poverty rate in Bali due to the fact that portion of the land is used for clove and coffee plantations. Thus, a large number of people leave their homes to find work in cities. Working aboard cruise ships or in the tourism industry in other cities in Bali Province is becoming increasingly popular among their working-age population.
4. Marapu

   Sumba Island is one of the islands in the province of East Nusa Tenggara (NTT) known as Tana Marapu or Bumi Marapu (Soeriadiredja, 2016), which administratively comprises the Districts of West Sumba, East Sumba, Southwest Sumba, and Central Sumba. The Marapu religion emerged and evolved in the Sumba Island region, and its adherents consider it to be the oldest religion that has existed on earth since the beginning of human life. In general, there are four sorts of social strata in Marapu society, all of which are determined by hereditary lines, particularly the male lineage (patrilineal).
5. Nuaulu

   The Nuaulu is one of the indigenous people dwelling on the mainland of "Nusa Ina" (Mother Island) or Seram Island in the Central Maluku District of Maluku

Province. The Nuaulu has its own unique culture and customs distinct from all other tribes on the Seram Island. The Nuaulu's indigenous peoples believe that a magical force known as Uppu Anahatana governs and controls their worldly lives. Although living near the coasts, most of the Nuaulu's peoples rely heavily on gardening and horticulture farming for their income.

6. Tugutil

   The Tugutil are an indigenous people who live in Halmahera Island in the eastern region of Indonesia, particularly in the province of North Maluku. The Tugutil people of East Halmahera District are the main subject of study in this book. Martodirdjo (1991: 97–98) said that "The Tugutil people are Tobelo-speaking residents known and living as forest dwellers in the northern and central parts of Halmahera Island." Today, the vast majority of them live a nomadic life deep in the interior forests or within the woods near the coast. Some others have begun living permanently with the locals near the beach, either on their own free will or as a result of government-sponsored relocation programs.

7. Orang Asli Papua

   Orang Asli Papua (The Indigenous Papuans) in this book refer to Biak indigenous communities. Biak-Numfor is also a region with a significant cultural history, such as the cargoist tradition and the legend of Manarmakari, which later spread to other regions, including Jayapura (Kamma, 1972). The Orang Asli Papua of Biak-Numfor share a collective history and memory of events from the past, such as the pandemics of Spanish flu and cholera in the late nineteenth century. They hold onto a belief system in which they recognize the presence of supernatural abilities referred to as "*fan nanggi*" and call their God who controls the cosmos as "*manseren nanggi.*" The Orang Asli Papua who live in urban areas are employed in the government bureaucracy, both civil and military, as teachers, medical personnel, priests, and in the economic sector as sellers of areca nut, noken, and fishery or agricultural products, whereas The Orang Asli Papua in rural or coastal areas are typically cultivators, copra producers, and fishermen.

The data in this book was collected using both qualitative and quantitative methods. In September 2021, in-depth interviews, Focus Group Discussions, and field observations on indigenous peoples in different locations were conducted to sustain the qualitative approach to the study. Indigenous peoples, local leaders, local governments, local and international NGOs, and academics were the key informants in each region. The quantitative data provided by the BPS-Statistics Indonesia, including the Population Census, Inter-Census Population Survey (SUPAS), National Labor Force Survey (Sakernas), and National Socio-Economic Survey (Susenas) were also used to support this book. These statistical data served not only as preliminary information, but also as an important material of analysis to establish qualitative findings.

1.5 Structure of the Book

This book is divided into four chapters, excluding the introduction and conclusion. It starts with Chapter 2, which examines indigenous peoples with a focus on Indonesia. This chapter will look deeper into the question of who Indonesia's indigenous populations are. In this chapter, indigenous peoples are discussed within two categories: ethical and emic. In the ethical category, attention is directed to theories and concepts of indigenous peoples in general as well as the researchers' point of view. Meanwhile, the emic category refers to the definition of indigenous peoples by the communities being studied, which is predominately based on similarities in cultural characteristics and ancestral beliefs.

Chapter 3 will address the vulnerability of indigenous peoples in seven sites across Indonesia. This chapter also deals with the COVID-19 pandemic, which has made many levels of society vulnerable. This chapter will elaborate on how to define and conceptualize the vulnerability, which is dynamic in nature, of indigenous peoples. In addition, the vulnerability of indigenous peoples in seven areas will also be examined in this section from various dimensions, including physical, ecological and health.

Chapter 4 looks at the impacts of the COVID-19 pandemic on indigenous communities in Indonesia, focusing on five aspects: fertility, mortality, health services, economy, and rituals. The changes that took place in the five aspects of impacts are recorded according to indigenous peoples' cultural perspectives in the seven locations. This chapter will also shed light on the unique features of indigenous peoples in various regions of Indonesia, thereby providing a wealth of information regarding the impacts that occur in their lives and livelihoods.

It is intriguing to examine various responses to the ongoing COVID-19 pandemic, particularly at the level of indigenous peoples (both individuals and communities) and the government. Chapter 5 will introduce the reader, first, to the local knowledge and culture of indigenous peoples in relation to the COVID-19 pandemic. Second, it will also highlight the adaption strategies in socioeconomic and cultural realms during the pandemic. Third, it will scrutinize the collaboration between indigenous peoples and local governments in fighting the pandemic. Indigenous peoples have been renowned for their richness of environmentally and ecologically responsible behaviors. In this pandemic era, medicines from nature become one of the primary sources; traditional lockdowns, which have been used for generations to protect against pandemics, are now back into the limelight. In addition, indigenous peoples' livelihoods that have shifted to services (such as tourism) receives attention for discussion in this chapter, elucidating how diversification of primary livelihoods such as agriculture, plantations, and fisheries becomes once again beacons of hope for survival.

This book contains a rich source of information from several indigenous communities in Indonesia, each with their own distinctive traits. Hopefully, this book will offer the readers with a comprehensive picture of how indigenous peoples in Indonesia have responded to the COVID-19 pandemic, either with their own methods and resources or with the aid of other parties. Thus, we will be able to learn a great deal from indigenous peoples in Indonesia about their strategies for coping with and adapting new traditions to the ongoing pandemic.

References

Andiarsi, M. K. (2020, October 10). Sebaran masyarakat adat. *kata data* https://katadata.co.id/padjar/infografik/5f803063 1f92a/sebaran-masyarakat-adat

Araujo, S., Cannon, M., Schmidt-Sane, M., Shankland, A., Snijder, M., & Wu, Y. C. (2021). Key considerations: Indigenous people in COVID-19 response and recovery. *Social Science in Humanitarian Action Platform*. https://www.socialscienceinaction.org/resources/key-considerations-indigenous-peoples-in-covid-19-response-and-recovery/

Asia-Pacific Economic Cooperation/ APEC. (2021). *Report: Understanding the economic impact of COVID-19 on indigenous peoples*. SOM Steering Committee on Economic and Technical Cooperation (SCE). https://www.apec.org/docs/default-source/publications/2021/10/understanding-the-economic-impact-of-covid-19-on-indigenous-peoples/221_sce_economic-impact-of-covid-19-on-indigenous-peoples.pdf?sfvrsn=76620920_1

Block, P., Hoffman, M., Raabe, I. J., Dowd, J. B., & Mills, M. C. (2020). Social network-based distancing strategies to flatten the COVID-19 curve in a post-lockdown world. arXiv: 2004.07052. https://doi.org/10.1038/s41562-020-0898-6

BPS (2020). Hasil survei sosial demografi dampak COVID-19. *Jakarta: Badan Pusat Statistik*. https://www.bps.go.id/id/publication/2020/06/01/669cb2e8646787e52dd171c4/hasil-surveisosial-demografi-dampak-covid-19-2020.html

Cardona, O. D., van Aalst, M. K., Birkmann, J., Fordham, M., McGregor, G., Perez, R., Pulwarty, R. S., Schipper, E. L. F., & Sinh, B. T. (2012). Determinants of risk: Exposure and vulnerability. In C. B. Field, V. Barros, T. F. Stocker, D. Qin, D. J. Dokken, K. L. Ebi, M. D. Mastrandrea, K. J. Mach, G.-K. Plattner, S. K. Allen, M. Tignor, & P. M. Midgley (Eds.), *Managing the risks of extreme events and disasters to advance climate change adaptation. A special report of working groups I and II of the Intergovernmental Panel on Climate Change (IPCC)* (pp. 65–108). Cambridge University Press. https://www.ipcc.ch/site/assets/uploads/2018/03/SREX-Chap2_FINAL-1.pdf

Chriscaden, K. (2020, Oktober 13). *Impact of COVID-19 on people's livelihoods, their health, and our food systems: Joint statement by ILO, FAO*. https://www.who.int/news/item/13-10-2020-impact-of-covid-19-on-people's-livelihoods-their-health-and-our-food-systems

Cord, L., & Pizarro, D. M. (2021, August 6). Indigenous Peoples' resilience: Supporting solutions from within. *World Bank Blog*. https://blogs.worldbank.org/voices/indigenous-peoples-resilience-supporting-solutions-within

Denny, D. M. T., Seixa, C., de Castro, D., & Pereira, L. I. (2021). COVID-19 magnifies the vulnerabilities: The Brazilian case. *International Journal of Discrimination and the Law, 21*(3), 272–287. https://doi.org/10.1177/13582291211031374

Dihni, V. A. (2021). Total kematian COVID-19 Indonesia peringkat ke-7 di dunia. *Katadata*. https://databoks.katadata.co.id/datapublish/2021/10/08/total-kematian-covid-19-indonesia-peringkat-ke-7-di-dunia

Economic Commission for Latin America and the Caribbean (ECLAC). (2021). *The impact of COVID-19 on indigenous peoples in Latin America (Abya Yala): Between invisibility and collective resistance*. Project Documents (LC/TS.2020/171). https://repositorio.cepal.org/bitstream/handle/11362/46698/S2000893_en.pdf?sequence=1

FAO. (2020, August 7). From the countryside with love: Combating food insecurity in Peru with ancestral solidarity during the COVID-19 crisis. *Food and Agriculture Organization of the United Nations*. https://www.fao.org/fao-stories/article/en/c/1300299/

Fineman, M. A. (2017). Vulnerability and inevitable inequality. *Olso Law Review, 4*, 133–149. https://doi.org/10.18261/issn.2387-3299-2017-03-02

Fineman, M. A. (2018). The vulnerable subject: Anchoring equality in the human condition. *Yale Journal of Law and Feminism, 20*(1). https://openyls.law.yale.edu/bitstream/handle/20.500.13051/6993/03_20YaleJL_Feminism1_2008_2009_.pdf?sequence=2

Fitzmaurice, M. (2021). The COVID-19 crisis, indigenous peoples, and international law: A vulnerability perspective. In M. M. Mbengue & J. D.'Aspremont (Eds.), *Crisis narratives in international law* (pp 173–181). https://doi.org/10.1163/9789004472365_019

Garrett, G. (2020, May 29). *The post-COVID-19 world will be less global and less urban.* Wharton Magazine. https://magazine.wharton.upenn.edu/digital/the-post-covid-19-world-will-be-less-global-and-less-urban/

GEF. (2020, August 7). Indigenous peoples and COVID-19: Response and resilience. *The GEF*. https://www.thegef.org/newsroom/blog/indigenous-peoples-and-covid-19-response-and-resilience

Gordon-Bouvier, E. (2021). Vulnerable bodies and invisible work: The COVID-19 pandemic and social reproduction. *International Journal of Discrimination and the Law, 21*(3), 212–229. https://doi.org/10.1177/13582291211031371

Huan, C., Ji, X., Zhou, W., Huang, Z., Peng, X., Fan, L., Ge, L., & Zhu, W. (2021). Coronavirus: A possible cause of reduced male fertility. *Andrology, 9*(1), 80–87. https://doi.org/10.1111/andr.12907

IFAD (2020, 29 December). A year in review: Nurturing resilient rural communities in a time of change. *IFAD*. https://www.ifad.org/en/w/news/a-year-in-review-nurturing-resilient-rural-communities-in-a-time-of-change

ILO. (2020). *Domestic violence and its impact on the world of work*. https://www.ilo.org/wcmsp5/groups/public/---dgreports/---gender/documents/briefingnote/wcms_738117.pdf

International Working Group for Indigenous Affairs (IWGIA). (2021). *The indigenous world 2021*. https://iwgia.org/doclink/iwgia-book-the-indigenous-world-2021-eng/eyJ0eXAiOiJKV1QiLCJhbGciOiJIUzI1NiJ9.eyJzdWIiOiJpd2dpYS1ib29rLXRoZS1pbmRpZ2Vub3VzLXdvcmxkLTIwMjEtZW5nIiwiaWF0IjoxNjE4OTE0NDcyLCJleHAiOjE2MTkwMDA4NzJ9.16jl03Uv-9UUBvvf4xV5yXkXCPlT46vbfKaGwvYvbvA

Jobe, K. S. (2021). The jurisprudence of universal subjectivity: COVID-19, vulnerability and housing. *International Journal of Discrimination and the Law, 21*(3), 254–271. https://doi.org/10.1177/13582291211032843

Kamma, F. C. (1972). *Koreri messianic movements in the Biak-Numfor culture area: Koninklijk Instituut Voor Taal-, Land-, En Volkenkunde Translation Series 15*. Springer Netherlands.

Kiwnuka, M. A. N. (2021). Institutional vulnerabilities, COVID-19, resilience mechanisms and societal relationships in developing countries. *International Journal of Discrimination and the Law, 21*(3), 88–307. https://doi.org/10.1177/13582291211031381

Leach, D. M., Baer, L. A., & Yu, P. (2020). Linking indigenous communities with regional development. *Organisation for Economic Cooperation and Development. The OECD Observer*, 1–3.

Martodirdjo, H. S. (1991). *Orang Tugutil di. Halmahera, struktur dan dinamika sosial masyarakat penghuni hutan*. [Disertasi Universitas Padjadjaran].

Milhorance, F. (2021, February 8). *Covid deaths of Yanomami children fuel fears for Brazil's indigenous*. The Guardian. https://www.theguardian.com/global-development/2021/feb/08/covid-deaths-yanomami-children-indigenous

Millalen, P., Nahuelpan, H., Hofflinger, A., & Martinez, E. (2020). COVID-19 and indigenous peoples in Chile: Vulnerability to contagion and mortality. *AlterNative: An International Journal of Indigenous Peoples, 16*(4), 399–402. https://doi.org/10.1177/1177180120967958

Nourgam, A. (2020). *Message from the chair of the permanent forum on indigenous issues to ensure indigenous peoples are informed, protected and prioritized during the global covid-19 pandemic*. Indigenous peoples and development branch/ secretariat of the permanent forum on indigenous issues Department of Economic and Social Affairs, United Nations.

Pitana, I. G. (1994). Desa adat dalam arus modernisasi. In I Gde Pitana (Eds.), *Dinamika masyarakat dan Kebudayaan Bali*. Penerbit BP.

Prasetijo, A. (2017). Living without the forest: Adaptive strategy of Orang Rimba. *Senri Ethnological Studies, 95* (Sedentarization among Nomadic Peoples in Asia and Africa), 255–278. https://doi.org/10.15021/00008586

Reuter, T. A. (2005). *Custodians of the sacred mountains: Budaya dan masyarakat di Pegunungan Bali*. Yayasan Obor Indonesia.

Satuan Tugas Penanganan COVID-19. (2022). Peta sebaran. https://covid19.go.id/peta-sebaran

Siriwardhane, P., & Khan, T. (2021). The gendered nature of the risk factors of the COVID-19 pandemic and gender equality: A literature review from a vulnerability perspective. *Sustainability, 13*(23), 13375. https://doi.org/10.3390/su132313375

Soeriadiredja, P. (2016). Tatanan hidup Orang Sumba (studi etnografis di Sumba Timur). Program Studi Antropologi, Fakultas Ilmu Budaya, Universitas Udayana, Denpasar.

Souisa, H., Wibawa, T., & Salim, N. (2020, May 28). *Indonesia is bracing for a coronavirus baby boom due to decline in contraceptive use, official says*. ABC NEWS. https://www.abc.net.au/news/2020-05-28/indonesia-predicts-coronavirus-baby-boom-hundreds-of-thousands/12286576

Steyn, N., Binny, R. N., Hannah, K., Hendy, S., James, A., Kukutai, T., Lustig, A., McLeod, M., Plank, M. J., Ridings, K., & Sporle, A. (2020). Estimated inequities in COVID-19 infection fatality rates by ethnicity for Aotearoa New Zealand. *The New Zealand Medical Journal, 133*(1520). https://doi.org/10.1101/2020.04.20.20073437

Ullah, M. A., Moin, A. T., Araf, Y., Bhuiyan, A. R., Griffiths, M. D., & Gozal, D. (2020). Potential effects of the COVID-19 pandemic on future birth rate. *Front. Public Health, 8*, 578438. https://doi.org/10.3389/fpubh.2020.57843

United Nations. (2020). *COVID-19 and indigenous peoples*. https://www.un.org/development/desa/indigenouspeoples/covid-19.html

Vishvkarma, R., & Rajender, S. (2020). Could SARS-CoV-2 affect male fertility? *Andrologia, 52*(9), Article e13712. https://doi.org/10.1111/and.13712

Walters, G., Broome, N., Cracco, M., Dash, T., Dudley, N., Elías, S., Hymas, O., Mangubhai, S., Mohan, V., Niederberger, T., Nkollo-Kema Kema, C. A., Oussou Lio, A., Raveloson, N., Rubis, J., Mathieu Toviehou, S. A. R., & Van Vliet, N. (2021). COVID-19, indigenous peoples, local communities and natural resource governance. *Parks, 27*, 57–62. https://doi.org/10.2305/IUCN.CH.2021.PARKS-27-SIGW.en

WHO (2020). Transmission of SARS-CoV-2: Implications for infection prevention precautions. *World Health Organization*. https://www.who.int/news-room/commentaries/detail/transmission-of-sars-cov-2-implications-for-infection-prevention-precautions

Wisner, B., Blaikie, P., Cannon, T., & Davis, I. (2004). *At risk: Natural Hazards, people's vulnerability and disasters*. Routledge.

Wordometer (2024, April 13). Coronavirus Death Toll. Accessed from Coronavirus Death Toll and Trends.

World Tourism Organization. (2021). *UNWTO inclusive recovery guide – Sociocultural impacts of COVID-19, Issue 4: Indigenous Communities*, UNWTO, Madrid. https://doi.org/10.18111/9789284422852

Chapter 2
Indigenous Peoples and Communities: A Conceptual Account

Cahyo Pamungkas, Muhammad Nur Prabowo Setyabudi, and Sari Seftiani

Abstract There are six subtitles in Chapter 2 to elaborate on the concept, definition, and category of indigenous peoples. Pamungkas et al. discuss the definition of ethnic groups and ethnicity in anthropology, followed by the distinctions between tribal communities and indigenous peoples in the second section. This part describes some definitions from various studies that are often used to see the indigenous peoples. Until now, anthropologists have referred to indigenous communities as tribes and indigenous peoples as ethnic groups. In the third section, the differences between indigenous customary peoples and indigenous peoples will be discussed. The fourth section describes the concept of local religion and belief-based indigenous peoples. Pamungkas et al. also show the categories of indigenous people that are conceptualized in the population census that registers indigenous peoples in Indonesia. In the last section, we classify indigenous peoples in this study based on numerous aspects of their daily life, including livelihoods, territories, and regions where they are living.

Keywords Indigenous people · Communities · Ethnic group · Ethnicity · Indonesia

As described in the preceding chapter, the subject of this study is a number of indigenous peoples who reside in several provinces in Indonesia. Due to the variety of indigenous peoples, there is also a spectrum of views in defining an indigenous group. Nongovernmental organizations such as The Indigenous Peoples' Alliance of

C. Pamungkas (✉)
Research Center for Area Studies, National Research and Innovation Agency (BRIN), Jakarta, Indonesia
e-mail: cahyo.pamungkas@brin.go.id

M. N. P. Setyabudi
Research Center for Society and Culture, National Research and Innovation Agency (BRIN), Jakarta, Indonesia

S. Seftiani
Research Center for Population, National Research and Innovation Agency (BRIN), Jakarta, Indonesia

C. Pamungkas et al. (eds.), *The Impact of the Pandemic on Indigenous People in Indonesia*, Quality of Life in Asia 20, https://doi.org/10.1007/978-981-96-4222-9_2

the Archipelago, for instance, defines indigenous peoples as a community that share the same culture and genealogy along with all of its resources, cultural traditions, and governance. The Directorate General of Culture includes local faith communities as part of tribal peoples (*masyarakat adat*). Whereas, several policies of the Central Government policies recognize only Indigenous Customary Communities (*Masyarakat Hukum Adat*) and not all indigenous peoples. Since there is no single definition of indigenous peoples, this section will examine those diverse perspectives, including the concept of indigenous peoples seen from anthropological lenses. Departing from the existing concepts, a new category of indigenous peoples will be built and developed based on the research conducted.

The first section will discuss the definition of ethnic groups and ethnicity in anthropology, followed by the distinctions between tribal communities and indigenous peoples in the second section. Until now, anthropologists have referred to indigenous communities as tribes and indigenous peoples as ethnic groups. In the third section, the differences between indigenous customary peoples and indigenous peoples will be discussed. The fourth section will describe the concept of local religion and belief-based indigenous peoples. In the concluding section, we will classify indigenous peoples in this study based on numerous aspects of their daily life, including livelihoods, territories, and regions where they are living.

2.1 The Conception of Ethnic Group and Ethnicity in Anthropology

We often hear the terms "indigenous people" and "tribal communities." What is the difference between the two, and can they both be thought of as ethnic groups and ethnicities? The following section attempts to explain what indigenous people and tribal communities are from a perspective of social anthropology. To define a term, one will certainly need a clear and relevant theoretical point of view. Thus, we will start with the basic idea of ethnic group and ethnicity.

In his book, *Rethinking Ethnicity*, Richard Jenkins (2008) discusses ethnicity through the lens of other scholars' perspectives on ethnic groups. Max Weber is one of them; he defines ethnic groups based on the shared beliefs of their members. According to Jenkins, based on Weber's perspective (1978), the commonality of cultural traits facilitates group formation only but does not determine the very structure of the group. Hughes (1994) argues that an ethnic group cannot be compared to other groups because it is bound by a set of social constraints that can be seen as "in" and "out" group boundaries. According to Hughes, ethnicity is what people believe about their cultural differences that become the markers of group membership.

In anthropology, definitions of ethnic groups and ethnicity can be traced back to the ideas of Fredrik Barth (1969). In a book that he edited, *Ethnic groups and Boundaries* he argued that ethnic groups had been so far defined according to reproductivity, shared basic cultural values, systems of interaction and communication (language) by which members of a group identify themselves or being identified by others. Barth does not deny the aforementioned cultural features, but he emphasizes that ethnic groups should be seen as a form of social organization. Ethnic groups are formed by the preservation of social boundaries through interactions between members of a group (us) and members of other groups (them). Defining ethnic groups is, therefore, a matter of establishing borders between us and them rather than cultural similarities. According to Koentjaraningrat (2004), the formation of an ethnic group is not only determined by shared cultural traits inherent in a group, but also recognition or ascription by other groups.

Since the 1960s, ethnic groups and ethnicity have been common terms in social anthropology and have been taken for granted without interrogating their meaning or context of application. Eriksen (2010) asserted that all anthropological perspectives concur that ethnicity is something related to classification of people and intergroup relations. Eriksen continued to explain that, in everyday life, ethnicity is associated with minorities and racial relations; however, in social anthropology, it refers to the features of intergroup relations in which individuals attribute themselves or being attributed by others as belonging to a certain group. In this situation, a minority group in a given country is no less ethnic than a majority group.

The term ethnic groups implies that there are intergroup links and relations and that we all live in a continuous world Talking about ethnic groups as social organizations living in complete isolation is absurd. An ethnic group or an ethnic category is created through intergroup interactions. A group's identity is always defined in relation to other groups.

Eriksen (2010) noted a shift from the term "tribe" to "ethnic group" that transcends the ethnocentric or Eurocentric bias that anthropologists have frequently used in their analysis of non-European countries. When we speak of a tribe or a community, we inadvertently impose a stark contrast between ourselves and the people we are studying and this generally correlates to the distinction between ethnic groups as a modern society and tribes as a traditional or primitive one. Thus, everyone, regardless of whether they live in Europe, Asia, North America, or the Pacific, is a member of an ethnic group although with different degrees of ethnic bonds.

Therefore, the following question is what differentiates one ethnic group from another ethnic group; are not they the same as human groups? Michael Moerman's study (1965) on the Lue ethnic group in Thailand can provide an answer when he tried to find out who the Lue people are and how they are distinguished from other ethnic groups. The anthropological perspective suggests that the boundaries of an ethnic group frequently refer to language, culture, politically organized practices, etc. Using this approach, he found no differences between the Lue people and other ethnic groups around as they share similar cultural characteristics. When he questioned the Lue what distinguishes them from other ethnic groups, he learned that their language, customs, and beliefs are virtually identical.

Moerman concluded that someone self-identifies as being a Lue because of the belief that the Lue call themselves as Lue people and act in ways that legitimize their Lue-ness. According to Moerman, this type of definition is an emic category of ascription, in which an ethnic category is defined by the ethnic group itself. From

Moerman's research findings we understand that ethnic groups do not always have cultures that are distinct from other groups, or that two ethnic groups with very similar identities can form two distinct ethnic groups. Thus, cultural similarities between the two groups is not a defining feature that defines an ethnic group. Similarly, two groups in Papua with different cultural traits in terms of language, belief, and technology, for example, do not always create interethnic interactions if they do not engage with one another. Eriksen (2010) explains as follows:

> Two distinctive, endogamous groups, say, somewhere in New Guinea, may well have widely different languages, religious beliefs and even technologies, but that does not necessarily mean that there is an ethnic relationship between them. For ethnicity to come about, the groups must have a minimum of contact with each other, and they must entertain ideas of each other as being culturally different from themselves. If these conditions are not fulfilled, there is no ethnicity, for ethnicity is essentially an aspect of a relationship, not a property of a group.

The key to defining an ethnic group is not the presence of cultural elements, but rather the occurrence of contact or interaction between groups that perceive themselves to be distinct. This approach, which is frequently referred to as interactionist definition of ethnicity, has been extensively explored by Fredrik Barth, Richard Jenkins, and Thomas H. Eriksen in contrast to the essentialist approach, which emphasizes cultural similarities in defining ethnic groups. Some groups seem to share similar cultural features, but their interethnic relations are conflictual. On the other side, within an ethnic group, there is also a degree of variation between its community members. How do we define the term "natives," who are sometimes referred to as "tribal communities" or "indigenous peoples" from an ethnicity-based perspective? Are they classified as ethnic or tribal groups?

2.2 Definition of Indigenous Peoples and Tribal Communities

Tribal communities or indigenous peoples are identical to peoples who are thought to be the original inhabitants in the territory of a state (Eriksen, 2010). Therefore, we begin with the most basic question: when did the term indigenous people first exist and when was the group internationally recognized? Considering that the terms ethnicity and ethnic groups were not commonly used until after World War II or the 1960s, the terms became part of scholarly discourse and policymaking. Even if anthropologists or legal experts from colonial countries, such as Van Volleh Hoven of the Netherlands, have defined indigenous peoples in the colonies, the existence of these societies remained a topic of debate at the United Nations until 1989. The terminology of "the native peoples" or "the indigenous peoples" were frequently contrasted with the sojourners or settlers, who were in most cases Western European immigrants in the colonies. How the discourse on indigenous peoples took place after the decolonization period, when some European immigrants had returned and others still dominated in various countries?

In 1989, the International Labor Organization (ILO) became the first international instrument to protect indigenous peoples by issuing the ILO Convention No. 169/1989. Article 2a of the Convention rejected the assimilationist approach to indigenous peoples and demanded the full realization of their social, economic, and cultural rights, as well as their social and cultural identities, customs and traditions, and institutions. As a result, national governments have begun abandoning strategies of forced assimilation; for instance, Australia's high court decided to acknowledge indigenous rights in the case of Mabo Landmark (Henley & Davidson, 2008). However, many countries have not yet ratified the treaty; only 17 of 160 countries have done so. In fact, Indonesia and a number of other Asian nations did not ratify it on the grounds that all ethnic groups living in Indonesia are indigenous, therefore there is no need to do so. This position is supported by Persoon (1998) and Li (2000), who argued that separating indigenous people from non-indigenous people is a hard subject. The majority of Asian countries, including Indonesia, make an assertions or a truism that nearly all Indonesians are indigenous as a rationale for rejecting the terminology of indigenous peoples while anticipating the ramifications of international debates. President Soeharto issued a policy that Indonesia is a nation without indigenous people or that all Indonesians are indigenous. The category of "indigenous and tribal peoples" that is defined and recognized in The ILO Convention 169 was considered to have no clear legal equivalent in Indonesia. Recognition of diversities in cultural groups in Indonesia always refers to the national emblem of *Bhinneka Tunggal Ika*, i.e., unity in diversity as reflected in the Taman Mini Indonesia Indah (TMII), which displays the notion that different cultures throughout the provinces are recognized. The development policies of The New Order and its successive regimes had been aimed to improve the fates of the ethnic groups or vulnerable people, notably those residing in rural and impoverished areas (Li, 2000).

According to Li (2000), the literal translations of indigenous people into original or native inhabitants are to some extent interchangeable. She argued that the international discourse on indigenous rights has influenced contemporary conceptualizations of custom (*adat*), particularly in terms of environmentalism and community-based natural resource management, introducing new ways of modeling, envisioning, and legitimizing communal lands and people's rights over the forest. According to Moniaga (1993) and Sangadji (1996), various publications by activists who struggle for the rights of indigenous people and who consistently refer to environmental politics, sustainability, and conservation have also contributed to this new development.

Referring to Li (2000), we can use the terms "indigenous people" and "ethnic peoples" interchangeably despite the fact that they have a different emphasis of meanings. Li (2000) pointed out that anthropologists in general rarely use the terms "tribe" or "ethnicity" to describe indigenous communities in Indonesia, while legal scholars continue to disagree about the use of "indigenous peoples" terminology, which is frequently situated within the colonial settings of social structure. The genealogical process by which an indigenous community or an indigenous people emerge is a central question frequently posed by anthropologists and scholars of customary law. Theoretically, Tania Li is of the opinion that the identification of a social group as an ethnic group, an indigenous group, or a native people has been never taken for granted, imposed, or created. Rather, it undergoes a process that is influenced by practices, landscapes, and meaning repertoires that have been historically deposited and inclusive of struggles within a given social formation. A no less important factor is the conjuncture in which some people self-identify as indigenous peoples in relation to how they renew their interactions with the nation, the government, and other ethnic groups in their immediate environment, all of which are products of agency and political articulation.

Articulation is a very important concept in defining a group referred to as indigenous peoples, which distinguishes them from tribal communities. Articulation contains the elements of struggle to gain recognition of identity and rights to land and natural resources from the state, the corporate, and the ethnic groups surrounding them. When a tribal community, with the intervention of non-governmental organizations, is fighting for recognition of its economic and sociocultural rights as guaranteed by the ILO Conventions, it might be referred to as "indigenous peoples." Therefore, the concept of articulation has distinguished "tribal or native communities" from "indigenous peoples" in which the latter is interchangeable with the term "ethnics" for the presence of contacts and interactions with other ethnics, the government or the corporate. According to an ethnicity perspective, the terminology of "ethnics" is produced through contacts and interactions to maintain social boundaries. If anthropologists moved from using the term "tribe" to "ethnic group" as explained in the previous discussion, there is also a similar shift in using the term "tribal communities" to "indigenous peoples." In ordinary life beyond the academic realm, however, the terms "tribal communities" and "indigenous peoples" are often confused.

Definitions of indigenous peoples as proposed by Tania Lie and the ideas of social boundaries formation as suggested by Barth, Jenkins, and Eriksen have been currently used in anthropological literatures. Semiarto Aji Purwanto, a professor of anthropology at the University of Indonesia (UI), for instance, wrote, "every indigenous group is a struggling group." Every native group is fighting for their economic and sociocultural rights against the dominance of government, industries, capitalism, and other forces that seek to subjugate their traditional culture for the sake of modernity and development. According to Purwanto (2021), globalization and modernization have brought changes into attitudes and viewpoints toward recognition of individual and collective identities.

The concept of modern humans grows concurrently with the expansion of capitalism, putting pressure on ethnic or socioeconomic groups that still adhere to their cultural traditions. Some of them are able to adapt to changes in the external environment and incorporate external values into their local cultures while maintaining the principles or norms of their time-honored traditions known as customs (*adat*). The alteration of traditional cultures cannot be separated from the shifts in the living space or ecological settings of tribal or indigenous peoples; the formerly hunting and farming grounds have now become concession areas for big plantations or modern mining operations. This development often results in the expropriation of lands belonging to indigenous communities or peoples, followed by a progressive loss of their natural resources and eventually their long-practice traditional values. Purwanto

(2021), quoting Van Wieren (2008) and Tanko (2020), exemplified that farming is not just an economic activity, but also a component of rituals tied to tradition and religious expression.

Thus, a shift in farming tradition to sedentary agriculture has consequently profound cultural ramifications. This has raised questions about the extent to which the government and civil societies pay attention to tribal communities and indigenous peoples in Indonesia. The terminology of the guidance of remote indigenous peoples (*pembinaan masyarakat adat terpencil*) used by the government in one of its initiatives demonstrates an etymological fallacy in defining indigenous peoples. Conceptually, indigenous peoples are civil society organizations struggling against the dominance of the state and industries; therefore, why should they be guided? Can this guidance be interpreted as an attempt to control indigenous peoples? The following section will elucidate the dynamics of the protection of indigenous communities in Indonesia.

2.3 Definition of Indigenous Peoples and Customary Law Peoples

As previously indicated, Indonesia and a number of Asian nations have not ratified the ILO convention protecting indigenous peoples. Since the 1998 reformation, however, the political discourse on the protection of indigenous peoples has begun to emerge along with the surge of democratization and political liberalization. During the New Order era, most human rights activists in Indonesia referred to the Basic Agrarian Law of 1960 (UUPA), which recognizes customary or traditional land rights. Thus, the term indigenous people or native people encompass not only a number of tribal groups living in remote places, but also most people dwelling in rural areas outside Java. They do not confine the definitions to the concept of customary law communities recognized by the Netherlands, but rather to the UUPA, so long as the lands stem from and are recognized by local traditions or customs (Li, 2000).

Zando Zakaria explained the discursive genealogy of indigenous peoples in Indonesia, which dates back to the Dutch period. The perspectives of customary law and ethnography in defining indigenous communities or people began to emerge during the colonial period. The viewpoints refer to Van Vollenhoven and can be divided into two major theories: customary law communities (*beschikkingrecht*) versus circles of customary communities (*rechtkringen*). According to the first theory, customary land rights (*ulayat*) are public, which means that the lands are still unsubdivided and jointly owned by all members of the community; nevertheless, they are also private in the sense that the lands have been shared to each family or individual. (i) When it comes to the public lands, the entities of customary law communities have the following authorities: rights of communities to the unworked lands, (ii) management of land utilization conducted by third parties, (iii) payment arrangements for land use by community members, (iv) community members' rights to regulate the cultivated lands, (v) collective territorial responsibility to outsiders, and (vi) permanence of community rights.

Customary Land Rights (*Hak Ulayat*) or Customary Territorial Rights (*Hak Wilayah Adat*) or whatever it is called are the ability of indigenous people to control, regulate, manage, utilize, and monitor a specific geographical and social area of land, water, and/or waters along with their natural within certain boundaries that have been set for generations (Sumardjono, 2005; Zakaria, 2021). As seen in the following table, customary land rights have various names in each area (Table 2.1).

The second theory refers to the circles of indigenous peoples or networks of communities known as traditional communities, not all of which can be called customary law communities because they depend on the possession of *ulayat* rights. According to Van Vollenhoven, there were nineteen indigenous community networks in the Dutch East Indies as follows:

1. Aceh (Aceh Besar, West Coast of Aceh, Singkil, Simeulue)
2. Gayo, Alas, and Batak
3. Minangkabau
4. South Sumatra (Bengkulu/Rejang, Lampung (Abung, Peminggir, Pubian, Rebang, Gedongtataan, Tulang Bawang), Palembang (Anak-Langitan, Jelma Daya, Kubu, Pasema, Semendo), Enggano
5. Malay (Lingga Riau, Indragiri, East Coast of North Sumatra, Banjar people)
6. Bangka and Belitung;
7. Kalimantan;
8. Minahasa
9. Gorontalo (Bolaang Mongondow, Boalemo);

Table 2.1 Names of *Ulayat* rights during the Dutch colonial period in the East Indies

No.	Home region/communities	Terminology	Meaning
1	Borneo	Penyampeto	The land that feeds
2	Bali	Prabumian	
3	Ambon	Petuanan	Tribal land
4	Borneo	Pewatasan	Limits of power
5	Ngada (Flores)	Ngora Gae	Ancestral land
6	Minangkabau	Ulayat	Territories
7	Java	Wewengkon	Ancestral land
8	Bolaang Mongondow	Tetabuan (tatabuan)	Forbidden to outsiders
9	Angkola	Torlok	
10	North Maluku	Abacocato	
11	South Sulawesi	Limpo	
12	Buru	Muru	
13	Central Lombok	Paer	Collective land rights

Source Zakaria (2021)

10. Tana Toraja (Central Sulawesi, Toraja, Baree-speaking Toraja, West Toraja, Sigi, Kaili, Tawaili, Toraja Sadan, To Mori, To Lainang, Banggai Islands of Indonesia)
11. South Sulawesi (Bugis, Bone, Laikang, Ponre, Mandar, Makassar, Selayar, Muna);
12. Ternate Islands
13. Maluku-Ambon
14. Irian/Papua
15. Timor Islands
16. Bali and Lombok
17. Central Java and East Java (including Madura)
18. Kingdom Area (Solo-Yogyakarta)
19. West Java (Parahyangan, Tanah Sunda, Jakarta, Banten)

Zakaria (2021) provides an illustration from the cultural region or circle of traditional Minangkabau society, which consists of two layers: the Minang people living outside their original lands (*perantauan*) and the Minang people settling in their hometown. There are four tiers of the Minang settlers: the *paruik*, the *kaum*, the *suku*, and the *nagari*. The *paruik* consists of all individuals who have blood relationship, i.e., having the same mother, whereas the *kaum* refers to all individuals bound by blood relationship of the clan, i.e., having the same grandmother. The *suku* is comprised of several clans with hereditary links, while the *nagari* is an alliance between tribes in a region. Customary law communities are found at the levels of the *kaum* and the *suku*, but not at the *nagari*, despite the fact that in the present days this sociocultural structure has changed significantly in accordance with the times.

In the legal system of Indonesia, the Constitutional Court No. 35/2012 established three basic criteria and requirements for the recognition of customary (law) communities. First, units of customary law communities and their traditional rights are known to be alive, whether geographically, genealogically, or functionally. This criterion requires that a unit of customary law community should have indigenous territory or rights (*ulayat*), the community members should share a sense of unity as a group, and it should have customary government structures, customary properties or objects, and a set of customary law standards. Second, a unit of customary law community and its traditional rights is considered in accordance with the development of society the indicator of which is its legal recognition under the laws applicable. Furthermore, the substance of its traditional rights is recognized and respected by the unit members and the larger communities and is not in contradiction with human rights. Third, a unit of customary law community along with its traditional rights should comply with the norms of the Unitary State of the Republic of Indonesia. The indicator is that it does not pose a threat to the integration of the Unitary State of the Republic of Indonesia, and that the substance of its customary law standards is consistent with and does not contradict the statutory provisions (Zakaria, 2021).

According to the Asian Development Bank, the international communities use the following more generic criteria: (i) Self-recognition and acceptance by others in the surroundings; (ii) The presence of collective attachments that geographically become a habitat separated from other groups and referred to as ancestral territories serving as a life sphere where the members make a living either intensively or seasonally; (iii) the availability of cultural, social, economic, political, and legal values and institutions different from those of other dominant groups; and (iv) occasionally the possession of language or, at the very least, a distinct dialect distinguishable from speakers of other languages and/or dialects. The second criterion is more cultural in the sense that it is applicable to indigenous people in general. Whereas, the first criterion is more legal-formal focusing on the customary law communities as defined by the government, which is in this case the Constitutional Court.

The Supreme Court's legal framework for recognition (Zakaria et al., 2020) has many drawbacks. It is too political, too bureaucratic, and too expensive to be compatible with socio-anthropological realities. The currently available policies exclusively target a single social unit with a private-public aspect, whereas in reality the lands and other natural resources are managed by diverse social units with only private authorities (family affairs in a broad sense). The political will of the Central Government for recognition is also relatively low. The solidity and self-regulating/self-governing capacity of society continue to decline or deteriorate because of regulations that do not provide certainty for the future, thereby leading to massive individualization.

2.4 Indigenous People and Local Religion or Belief

If we delve deeper into indigenous peoples as defined by AMAN (Zakaria 2021) and by the Constitutional Court (2012), we find that their definitions focus solely on the aspects of territories, genealogy, customary lands, shared group feelings, customary governance institutions, customary properties, and legal norms. However, in daily activities there are indigenous peoples based on local faiths, such as the Sunda Wiwitan, the Samin, the Tengger, and others who believe in God Almighty. In fact, not all of these groups had customary territories, hence they do not fit the aforementioned classification.

In addition to customary institutions, religious systems or beliefs cannot be separated from the existence of indigenous peoples. Local belief is typically not a separate component of local culture, but rather an integrated part of it. This is especially evident when referring to the traditional understanding of *adat* as a whole unit of customs, traditions, laws, and religion, and hence *adat* and religion are inseparable. Indigenous people embrace religious ideas and manifestations that differ from those of mainstream religions. While the latter is described as formal religions and is identified with revealed religion in religious studies, the former refers to bottom-up beliefs that emerge naturally (natural religion) and spread across various indigenous peoples and later become known as local or ancestral religion (*agama leluhur*). It is often that the political-administrative governance of religion only acknowledges the former and not the latter. Nevertheless, from an intellectual standpoint, religion encompasses revealed religion, natural religion, and local religion. In Indonesia, indigenous religion is politically and administratively denoted as "belief (*kepercayaan*)" or in a full name "belief in God Almighty (*kepercayaan kepada Tuhan YME*)," while other experts refer to it as "ancestral religion." There is no single term for local beliefs intrinsic to indigenous peoples, and their identities are likewise diverse, although the term "local religion (*agama lokal*)" is widely used in reference to the origin of its growth and the scope of its spread.

In social anthropology, religion is viewed through its cultural manifestations and is defined as a cultural system. In the words of scholars such as Thomas O'dea, religion or *religare* refers to aspects of faith and rituals within a communal group, being expressed in the belief that something transcendental exists above or beyond the range of human sense but nevertheless holds a very important position because it embodies the innermost desires of mankind and becomes the fountainhead of a given civilization (Marzali, 2016: 59).

Some scholars, including Melford Spiro, define religion as "an institution consisting of culturally patterned interaction with culturally postulated superhuman beings." Institution in this context does not refer to formal organizations, but rather to "socially shared patterns of action and belief" (Marzali, 2016: 60).

A symbolic interpretation of religion is found in Clifford Geertz's definition: "a system of symbols which acts to establish powerful, pervasive, and long lasting moods and motivations in men by formulating conceptions of a general order of existence and clothing these conceptions with such an aura of factuality that the moods and motivations seem uniquely realistic." Religion is a symbolic system with psychological, cultural, and social functions because of which moods and motivations seem to be factually true. Geertz's definition represents a symbolic and functional approach to religion (Marzali, 2016: 61).

Another scholar, Milton Yinger (1957), defines religion as something cultural: "religion is the cultural knowledge of the supernatural that people use to cope with the ultimate problem of human existence." Yinger emphasizes that religion is a cultural understanding of the supernatural that humans utilize to deal with the most critical question about human's existence on earth. Religion in essence is cultural knowledge and therefore is seen as human rather than divine creation (Marzali, 2016: 61). Graham Harvey holds the same view that religion is a human strategy to achieving what makes life happier, better, and healthier; for this reason humans are not only observing God's commands but also creating structures and efforts through which they perform specific rituals, activities, and reciprocal or hierarchical relationships. Harvey (2000) wrote, "Religions are human activities. Humans approach that which is of considerable, and sometimes ultimate, significance for them, by means of ceremonies, identification, and other expressions of reciprocal or hierarchical relationships."

Other substantive definitions see religion as a belief in supernatural beings or forces. Thus, the primary components of religion are rituals and beliefs. In contrast to theologians, social anthropologists define religion from a substantive and symbolic-functional standpoint by putting more stress on the aspects of rituals and rituals.

From this general concept of religion, we will explore in greater detail how local religions, which can be viewed socially anthropologically as beliefs and religions with distinct articulations and rites, are strongly, although not necessarily, rooted in indigenous and ethnic communities to the extent it has been commonly referred to as ethnic or local religions as opposed to official religions. In terms of meaning, local religions are closer to indigenous religions than global religions. In the still dualistic political-administrative religious framework, local religions are administratively under the auspices of the ministry of education and culture rather than the ministry of religion. Indonesia is home to more than 1,300 ethnic groups, each with distinct religious identities, traditions, and beliefs.

In terms of numbers, according to Graham Harvey (2000: 3), indigenous or local religions constitutes the majority of religions in the world due to their incredibly diverse number in almost every country; however, in terms of adherents and recognition, they are a minority and even marginal compared to global religions. It is quite often that local religions are inherently attributed to indigenous peoples and local communities. In addition, scholars typically divide them into two types. The first is a local religion that has survived and developed for centuries in a specific geographic community or setting. The second is a local religion whose devotees have spread it to other regions, mixing it with aspects of mainstream religions and thus no longer fully genuine.

This polarization occurs because religion is dynamic in nature. The rise and development of global religions lead to the elimination of customs and traditions-based religions; some of them even have been already extinct. Their number is insignificant when compared to adherents of major religions. However, the opposite is true when looking at their total number, which is approximately 299,617 (BPS, 2013). Then later in development local religions are rejected or even eradicated along with the domination of major religions. Some are then blended and mixed with components of major religions; others are extinct, and still others bring up creativity of new syncretic religions. There are also some believers who later become active in a traditional religion while simultaneously adopting a new religion (Harvey, 2000: 4).

According to international standards, the concept of "local beliefs" refers to values and spiritual practices inherent to those who are designated as "local communities" under international law, which are defined as:

> Indigenous communities, peoples and nations are those which, having a historical continuity with pre-invasion and pre-colonial societies that developed on their territories, consider themselves distinct from other sectors of the societies now prevailing on those territories, or parts of them. They form at present non-dominant sectors of society and are determined to preserve, develop and transmit to future generations their ancestral territories, and their ethnic identity, as the basis of their continued existence as peoples, in accordance with their own cultural patterns, social institutions, and legal system. (United Nations, 2004)

Local religion is understood as a culture in general, or a more specific manifestations of culture (Tuhri, 2020) in which religion is explained to be a factor of historical bonds for an ethnic group. Tuhri said,

> This historical continuity may consist of the continuation, for an extended period reaching into the presence of one or more of the following factors: ...Culture in general, or in specific manifestations (such as religion, living under a tribal system, membership of an indigenous community, dress, means of livelihood, lifestyle, etc.). (Tuhri, 2020)

Thus, seen from the international definition of religion above, the ideas of "indigenous peoples" or "traditional local communities" include religious beliefs as cultural expressions.

In Indonesia, almost all of the nineteen indigenous community networks that Van Vollenhoven listed above—despite criticism from other scholars over his classification and categorization for their shortcomings—have ties to local religious or ethnic beliefs. Some of those groups are easily identifiable, while others are not; some have gone extinct because of failed preservation or political policies in the past. A number of local religions have survived among indigenous communities in Indonesia, including the local religion of Adam, the beliefs of the Samin or Wong Sikep, and an indigenous peoples who live in the interior areas of Blora, Pati, Grobogan, Kudus, Central Java, and Bojonegoro, East Java. Another example is the belief of the Agama Djawa Sunda (ADS) found in the territories of the Sundanese indigenous peoples in West Java, which is often associated also with the Sunda Wiwitan or Adat Karuhun Urang (AKUR). In other parts of Sumatra, the Dayak people belong to the local religion of Malim or Ugamo Malim even before, they believe, Islam or Christianity came to their lands. The indigenous people of Toraja in South Sulawesi adhere to an ancestral religion called Aluk Todolo, which is known also as Alukta. Meanwhile, the Dayak people of Kalimantan uphold their ancestral religion named the Kaharingan. Apart from those mentioned above, there are many other local religions among various indigenous peoples (see Burhani & Sila, 2021).

Thus, indigenous peoples are indispensable from their religions or beliefs. In addition to following their customary laws, indigenous leaders often hold an authority to lead religious rituals, because of which people listen to them. In the Tengger indigenous peoples, who follow the original Javanese Buddhist religion of Sanyata, such religious authority belongs to a shaman who knows special spells and is believed to be a mediator between the underworld (the real world) and the upper world (the imaginary or supra-empirical world where ancestral spirits live) and lead every traditional ritual.

In Indonesia's Population Census, local religious groups of a given ethnicity are put into a category of "other religions (*agama yang lain*)" in addition to the five recognized religions. The 2010 Population Census recorded that they made up about 0.13% of Indonesia's population, but this number only came from fifteen largest ethnic groups in Indonesia. This means that in theory local religions of ethnic groups are recognized, and in practice, the average ethnic groups in Indonesia are the followers of religions even though they are outside of the recognized religions. This number is likely to rise as more people are becoming aware of their rights to religious freedom (Ananta et al, 2015: 271).

2.5 Indigenous Peoples as Conceptualized in the 2020 Population Census

The population censuses conducted by The Central Bureau of Statistics include "indigenous peoples" into the category of an ethnic-nation groups (*suku bangsa*). An ethnic-nation group is defined as a group that has been established for generations. As part of community cultural systems, the identity and attributes of an ethnic-nation group are inherited from generation to generation and are inherent in any individual following his or her parents' ethnic "identity."

In the 2010 and 2020 Population Censuses, one's ethnic-nation is identified according to a paternalistic line, which refers to the origins of the father's lineage. Nevertheless, there are some ethnic-nation groups in Indonesia who identify themselves based on the mother's bloodline, or maternalistic lineage, such as the Minang ethnic-nation group. The enumeration of ethnic-nation somehow incorporates the subjective elements other than lineage, therefore there is a need to take into account the informants' ideas and recognition. Thus, the primary concern in ethnic-nation identity lies in one's biological ties, especially those of "genuine" descent from the father's or mother's bloodlines, as well as the "articulation" of one's meaning and interactions.

In determining ethnicity, the enumeration was carried out in three stages of classification. First, the BPS used a location-based strategy due to the fact that an ethnic-nation, besides pointing to the origins of descendants by which a community unit is established, also encompasses the concept of a community unit dwelling in a certain geographic or administrative area, simultaneously showing the origin of an ethnic-nation group. Accordingly, the BPS mapping resulted in a classification of seven island regions as rings of ethnic-nation communities: Sumatra, Java and Bali, Nusa Tenggara, Kalimantan, Sulawesi, Maluku, and Papua. The Bataks, for example, are an ethnic group that historically originated in the Sumatran region. In the later stage, the mapping categorized each ethnic-nation group into the environment of the region, which reveals the origins of each ethnic group.

At a later stage, a family of ethnic-nation is more specifically categorized into a certain ethnic-nation group. The Bataks, for example, includes the Mandailing Batak, the Toba Batak, and so on. When it is not possible to identify which ethnic family a certain ethnic-nation group belongs to, the given group will be classified as a separate ethnic-nation provided that its population exceeds one million individuals; otherwise, it will be incorporated into a different ethnic group. For example, the ethnic groups of Sulawesi is a combination of 208 small ethnic groups in addition to the Makasarese, Bugis, Minahasa, and Gorontalo. According to the 2010 Population Census, the total number of ethnic groups in Indonesia is more than 1300 ethnic-nation groups with varying characteristics, populations, and living areas. Based on this classification method, the existing ethnic-nation groups were categorized into thirty-one major ethnic-nation groups. The Javanese are the largest ethnic-nation group spreading in nearly all Indonesian territories, with a population of 95.2 million peoples or 40% of Indonesia's total population. The Sundanese (36.7 million) and the Bataks (8.5

million) are the next three largest ethnic-nation groups in Indonesia. On the other hand, the Nias (1.04 million people), the Minahasa (1.24 million people), and the Gorontalo (1.25 million people) are ethnic-nation groups with the smallest population numbers (BPS, 2010).

However, the BPS classification of ethnicity has drawn criticism and feedback for containing flaws in its coding process for ethnic categories in which multiple categories are integrated into one ethnic category, thereby diminishing the diversities in the field as well as the informants' agency to establish their own ethnic classification. It is important for the researchers to have the necessary expertise to classify ethnic groups. In addition, contacts between people from different backgrounds should be also expected, which will likely increase the proportion of people who identify themselves with more than one ethnicity, not only with their ancestry-based ethnicity. The same is also true for classification of local religions or beliefs. Democracy should afford everyone the greatest opportunity to express their thoughts and beliefs (Ananta et al., 2015: 14).

So far, the enumeration in Indonesia is limited only to include the diversity of local religions inherent in ethnic life into the category of "other religions." But this category has multiple interpretations, whether it includes local or indigenous religions, other global religions such as Bahai or Sikh, or no religion at all. Therefore, Aris suggested that in the context of future democratization, any enumeration and survey should extend to the smallest category such as denominations that develop within ethnic groups in Indonesia; by doing so, they will be able to demonstrate the statistical significance of ethnicity and gain a better understanding of the spread of religion and spirituality within indigenous peoples and societies in general (Ananta et al., 2015: 14).

2.6 The Category of Society Being Studied

For the purposes of this study, we divided indigenous peoples into four groups:

Territory-based indigenous peoples: Orang Rimba, Tugutil, Nuaulu, Orang Asli Papua, and Tengger

Religion-based indigenous peoples: Marapu, Bali Aga, and Tengger

Livelihood-based indigenous peoples:

- Farming and hunting (Orang Rimba, Nuaulu, Orang Asli Papua, Tugutil)
- Tourism—Micro, Small, and Medium-Scale Business or UMKM (Orang Asli Papua, Bali Aga, Marapu)
- Agriculture and Fisheries (Orang Asia Papua, Tengger)

Region-Based Indigenous Peoples:

- Village: (Orang Rimba, Tengger, Tugutil, Nuaulu)
- City: (Bali Aga, Orang Asli Papua in Biak)
- Islands: (Orang Asli Papua in Padaido Islands)

This study employs the term "indigenous peoples" rather than "tribal communities" and "customary law communities" given that all of the indigenous populations we examined have been interacting with modernity and have not been living in isolation from the outer world. In addition, the category of indigenous peoples is much broader in scope than that of customary law communities whose presence require indigenous territories. Not all of the indigenous peoples we studied has had traditional lands recognized by the Government despite their ancestral land claims. In addition, some of our research subjects are being tied as indigenous peoples based more on local religions or beliefs. This study demonstrates that there is no single definition that can classify all of indigenous peoples, especially in Indonesia.

Based on the previous definitions that divide indigenous peoples into two categories: territorial and genealogical units and local religions or beliefs, we come up with two types of indigenous peoples. The first is territory and genealogy-based indigenous peoples, such as the Rimbas, the Tugutils, the Papuas, the Nuaulus, and the Tenggers. They are communities who believe to have originated from the same ancestor, have inhabited a region for generations, and have had their own customary territories, resources, norms, and system of governance. The second is religion-based indigenous peoples who consist of the Bali Aga, the Marapu, and the Tengger. The Bali Aga is bound by a unit of people belonging to the native Hindu, not the Majapahit Hindu inherited by the Tengger people. Whereas, the Marapu are the people who embrace a type of local religion that has been present prior to the arrival of Catholicism on Sumba Island.

In their daily lives, the indigenous peoples we studied engage in a variety of occupations, ranging from agriculture to "industries," according to the field data. Based on their primary livelihoods, the indigenous peoples are divided into four categories. The first is indigenous peoples who subsist on swidden cultivation and hunting, for which the Orang Rimba, Jambi and the indigenous Papuans of Biak are the examples. They plant tubers on constantly yet not-too-far shifting terrains and still hunts forest animals. However, over times it becomes difficult for them to hunt since their forests has been taken over by companies or the prey animals has been completely gone. The second is indigenous peoples who rely on sedentary agriculture and fishing for a living. This classification applies to the indigenous Papuans—who have begun farming commercial crops such as ginger, vegetables, and fruits and capturing fish with modern technologies—and the Tenggerese who work in agriculture. The third is indigenous peoples who make a living from the cultural tourism sector as small and medium-sized business owners producing souvenirs or maintaining tourist attractions in their areas. It includes the indigenous Papuans, the Bali Aga, and the people of Marapu. We also found the fourth category, which refers to indigenous peoples working in the smallholder industry sector, particularly the coffee, sago, and copra processing industries. Albeit in small numbers, we were able to find this group as part of the indigenous Papuan people of Biak.

Finally, our research also found the diversity of indigenous peoples based on their living areas or the ecological habitat wherein they survive and develop. Most of the indigenous peoples we met live in rural areas or in the middle of the forest, such as the Rimbas, the Tenggers, the Nuaulus, the Tugutils and the native Papuans. Some live in the urban areas, such as the Bali Aga in the province of Bali and the native Papuans in Biak. Only some native Papuans, who became the subject of our study, live in the islands, namely the Padaido Islands in Biak and the Numfor Island. This diversity of ecological habitats has more or less shaped their response to the pandemic. For example, the indigenous peoples in the islands suffer from transportation restrictions and the low price of fish so they start working as copra makers. Whereas, the indigenous peoples in the rural areas are relatively unaffected because they return to the agricultural sector, working more diligently in the plantations that was abandoned prior to the pandemic. More stories on the lives of indigenous peoples during the pandemic will be presented in the following chapters of this book.

References

Ananta, A., Arifin, E. N., & Hasbullah, M. S. (2015). *Demography of Indonesia's ethnicity*. ISEAS Publishing.
Barth, F. (1969) Ethnic groups and boundaries. *Little, Brown.*
BPS BALI (ini untuk tabel).
BPS (2010). Kewarganegaraan, Suku Bangsa, Agama, dan Bahasa Sehari-Hari. https://www.bps.go.id/id/publication/2012/05/23/55eca38b7fe0830834605b35/kewarganegaraan-suku-bangsa-agama-dan-bahasa-sehari-hari-penduduk-indonesia
Burhani, A. N. & Sila, M. A. (2021). *Agama, kepercayaan, dan paham Keagamaan.* Badang Libtang dan Diklat Kemenag RI.
Constitional Court (2012). Putusan MK 35/2012 tentang Hutan Adat sebagai hutan negara. Accessed on Microsoft Word-35-PUU-X-2012-ok.
Eriksen, T. H. (2010). *Ethnicity and nationalism: Anthropological perspectives.* Pluto Press.
Harvey, G. (2000). *Indigenous religions: A companion.* Cassell.
Henley, D., & Davidson, J. S. (2008). In the Name of Adat: Regional Perspectives on Reform, Tradition, and Democracy in Indonesia. *Modern Asian Studies, 42*(4), 815–852. https://doi.org/10.1017/S0026749X07003083
Hughes, E. C. (1994). *On work, race and the sociological imagination.* In L. A. Coser (Ed.), University of Chicago Press.
Jenkins, R. (2008). Rethinking ethnicity. SAGE.
Koentjaraningrat. (2004). Kebudayaan, Mentalitet dan Pembangunan. Jakarta: Gramedia.
Li, T. M. (2000). Articulating indigenous identity in Indonesia: Resource politics and the tribal slot. *Comparative Studies in Society and History, 42*(1), 149–179. https://doi.org/10.1017/S0010417500002632
Marzali, A. (2016). Agama dan kebudayaan. *Umbara, Indonesian Journal of Anthropology, 1*(1).
Moerman, M. (1965). Ethnic identification in a complex civilization: Who are the lue?. *American Anthropologist, 67*(5), 1215–1230. https://doi.org/10.1525/aa.1965.67.5.02a00070
Moniaga, S. (1993). The systematic destruction of the indigenous system of various adat communities throughout Indonesia. In H. P. Arimbi (Ed.), *Proceeding, seminar on the human dimensions of environmentally sound development* (pp. 31–36). WALHI and Friends of the Earth.
Persoon, G. (1998). Isolated groups or indigenous peoples: Indonesia and the international discourse. *Bijdragen tot de Taal-, Land-en Volkenkunde, 154*(2), 281–304. https://doi.org/10.1163/22134379-90003899
Purwanto, S. A. (2021). Kebijakan Budaya; Upaya Mengembangkan Komunitas dan Budaya Nusantara (Pidato Pengukuhan Guru Besar Antropologi). November), 0–20.
Sangadji, A. (1996). Menyorot PLTA Lore Lindu. *Palu: Yayasan Tanah Merdeka.*

Sumardjono, M. S. (2005). *Tanah dalam perspektif hak ekonomi sosial dan budaya*. Kompas Media Nusantara.
Tanko, M. (2020). Is farming a belief in Northern Ghana? Exploring the dual-system theory for commerce, culture, religion and technology. *Technology in Society 63*. https://doi.org/10.1016/j.techsoc.2020.101339
Tuhri, M. (2020). Religion and land rights in Indonesian Indigenous–State relations (Case Study of Orang Rimba in Jambi). *Religió: Jurnal Studi Agama-agama, 10*(2), 230–251. https://doi.org/10.15642/religio.v10i2.1386
United Nations. (2004). *The concept of indigenous peoples*. Department of economic and social affairs. Division for social policy and development secretariat of the permanent forum on indigenous issues.
Van Wieren, G. (2008). Ecological restoration as public spiritual practice. *Worldviews, 12*(2–3), 237–254. https://doi.org/10.1163/156853508X360000
Weber, M. (1978). *Economy and society: An outline of interpretive sociology*. In G. Roth & C. Wittich (Eds.), University of California Press.
Yinger, J. M. (1957). The Scientific Study of Religion. Macmillan Publishing.
Zakaria, Y., Iswari, P., Simarmarta, R., & Suprapto, E. (2020). potensi integrasi hutan adat ke dalam sistem verifikasi legalitas kayu (SVLK). KARSA dan European Forest Institute (EFI).
Zakaria, Y. (2021). Dinamika pengakuan dan perlindungan hak masyarakat adat dalam tatanan masyarakat Indonesia yang majemuk [visiting lecture]. Fakultas Ilmu Sosial dan Politik, Universitas Airlangga Surabaya.

Chapter 3
Indigenous Peoples' Vulnerability and the Pandemic: Between Capacity and Sensitivity

Gusti Ayu Ketut Surtiari, Abdul Fikri Angga Reksa, Hardianto, Risyanto, and Rachmi Agustiyani

Abstract This chapter provides a more comprehensive account of vulnerability since it considers the pandemic situation, which has created a massive disruption in this century. This chapter contains two major sections, both with a profound meaning: indigenous peoples and vulnerability. There has been no definite definition of indigenous people, and its related concepts and terminology are used all in a dynamic way depending on the context and time. The same applies to vulnerability, a term that is still open to being redefined. Due to the very diverse and unique conditions of indigenous peoples in each research site, this study uses the concept of relative vulnerability with a focus on its dynamic process. For instance, one indigenous people may not be as vulnerable as others in a specific period of time. In a similar manner, their vulnerability may change after they have taken measures or received an intervention. In general, Surtiari et al. distinguish two basic indicators of vulnerability: cognitive and quantitative measurements. The first refers to perceptions toward the COVID-19 pandemic, while the second includes socio-demographic aspects. In the field research conducted in Bali, Central Maluku (Maluku), Jambi, North Halmahera (North Maluku), Sumba (East Nusa Tenggara), and Malang (East Java), we highlighted seven measurable characteristics that have a crucial role in

G. A. K. Surtiari (✉) · A. F. A. Reksa · R. Agustiyani
Research Center for Population, National Research and Innovation Agency (BRIN), Jakarta, Indonesia
e-mail: gust003@brin.go.id

A. F. A. Reksa
Research Center for Area Studies, National Research and Innovation Agency (BRIN), Jakarta, Indonesia

Hardianto
Lampung Province, BPS-Statistics Indonesia, Bandar Lampung, Indonesia

Risyanto
Research Center for Social Welfare, Village, and Connectivity, National Research and Innovation Agency (BRIN), Jakarta, Indonesia

R. Agustiyani
Directorate of Population and Manpower Statistics, BPS-Statistics Indonesia, Jakarta, Indonesia

C. Pamungkas et al. (eds.), *The Impact of the Pandemic on Indigenous People in Indonesia*, Quality of Life in Asia 20, https://doi.org/10.1007/978-981-96-4222-9_3

estimating the vulnerability of an area or population to the COVID-19 pandemic. The socio-demographic categories consist of age group, gender, population mobility, health behavior, settlement patterns, livelihoods, and sociocultural activities.

Keywords Indigenous people · COVID-19 pandemic · Vulnerability · Capacity · Sensitivity

Indigenous peoples' vulnerability during the COVID-19 has not much received attention from scholars, whereas it is important to explore it in order to enhance the concept of vulnerability that has been established over the past three decades. The current Chapter will provide a more comprehensive account of vulnerability since it takes into account the pandemic situation, which has created a massive disruption in this century. This Chapter contains two major sections, both with a profound meaning: indigenous peoples and vulnerability. There has been no definite definition of indigenous peoples and its related concepts and terminology are used all in a dynamic way depending on the context and time. The same applies to vulnerability, a term that is still open to be redefined. Due to the very diverse and unique conditions of indigenous peoples in each research site, this study uses the concept of relative vulnerability with a focus on its dynamic process. For instance, one indigenous people may not be as vulnerable as others in specific period of time. In a similar manner, their vulnerability may change after they have taken measures or received an intervention.

In this study, vulnerability is defined as an individual's or a group's predisposition or propensity to experience a certain degree of calamity, loss, and damage when one or more specific dangers occur (Wisner et al., 2004). Vulnerability encompasses the susceptibility or sensitivity of system elements that exist within a community, as well as coping and adaptive methods for preventing or responding to a threat or an actual occurrence of hazard, including to avert a wider exposure. Furthermore, vulnerability is multidimensional, as it incorporates several institutional, economic, social, political, and environmental factors and is subject to the influence of interconnections across temporal and spatial scales (Cardona et al., 2012). It is important to note that in this section capacity and sensitivity serve as two primary components of vulnerability and will become a point of discussion.

Looking at the evolution of its concept and definition, vulnerability as a concept was initially rooted geography and natural disaster studies but it has since spread to various scientific fields, including development studies, particularly on the topic of poverty (Sen, 1981; Chambers, 1989; Dutta et al., 2011), public health sciences, medicine, sociology, psychology, humanity, and food safety. Since the 1990s, vulnerability has been widely used and developed to explain the specific conditions of individuals or communities prone to bear the harmful impacts of climate change (Adger, 2006). Different concepts have been used to describe vulnerability, showing that its definition will always change according to when, where, and under which context it occurs. Vulnerability should not be gauged merely on the basis of observable indicators like socio-demographic variables; it is also essential to measure vulnerability from a cognitive perspective, namely perception (Garschagen, 2014).

It is important to clarify the applicability of the concept of vulnerability in the context of the COVID-19 pandemic. Who are the vulnerable groups and why and how they become vulnerable are crucial questions that need to be answered. Bohle's concept (2001) becomes a relevant departure to define the concept of vulnerability, for it does not rest alone on quantitatively measurable indicators or variables. Bohle (2001) propounded a double structural vulnerability that looks at both internal and external aspects of vulnerability. On the internal aspect, an emphasis is laid on the capacity of an individual or a group to withstand the effects of current dangers. Although it is not explicitly mentioned how perception shapes internal abilities, the later development of this concept suggests that a person's perception for hazards will determine what the responses will be (Canon, 2015). Therefore, redefining vulnerable groups is of great importance, particularly during the current pandemic (Lancet, 2020) because a person who was not considered vulnerable at the onset of the pandemic could become extremely vulnerable and depend heavily on the responses from the government. The risk of suddenly loosing income or access to social supports has unimaginable repercussions, making it uneasy to identify all of those who may be vulnerable.

Obviously, the concept of vulnerable groups in the midst of the COVID-19 pandemic encompasses people from various socioeconomic classes struggling to survive financially, mentally, or physically during times of crisis. A valuable lesson learned from the pandemic is that a person's or group's perspective of the pandemic, either directly or indirectly, affects their sensitivity to economic and health repercussions. As an example, there are some groups of people who do not believe that a pandemic poses a threat to their lives; they seek to live a regular life while adhering to their ancestors' healthy living practices, such as taking traditional herbs to maintain a healthy body. On the basis of these facts, it is necessary to conduct more in-depth and comprehensive studies on the vulnerability of individuals and groups, particularly indigenous peoples.

Several studies have shown that indigenous peoples are vulnerable to the impacts of the COVID-19 pandemic (Niko, 2020). As described in Chapter One, indigenous peoples are classified as vulnerable groups if the concept used is vulnerability measured from the indicators of access to health care, information, and other public amenities. Some facts show that indigenous peoples in Indonesia are lacking access to reliable information during the pandemic, hence many of them do not know the best ways to prepare. Inadequate access to health care and the absence of social security also contribute to indigenous peoples' increased vulnerability (Power et al., 2020). In the context of indigenous peoples in Indonesia, there are in fact individuals who still do not have residential identity cards (KTP) and hence cannot receive social assistance programs. Nonetheless, if one considers some of their local wisdoms, such as the elders' orders to restrict interaction with outsiders and consume traditional herbs, indigenous peoples do have internal mechanisms that help strengthen their resilience to the pandemic.

In general, this chapter distinguish two basic indicators of vulnerability: cognitive and quantitative measurements. The first refer to perceptions toward the COVID-19 pandemic, while the second includes socio-demographic aspects. In the field researches conducted in Bali, Central Maluku (Maluku), Jambi, North Halmahera (North Maluku), Sumba (East Nusa Tenggara), and Malang (East Java), we highlighted seven measurable characteristics that have a crucial role in estimating the vulnerability of an area or population to the COVID-19 pandemic. The socio-demographic categories consist of age group, gender, population mobility, health behavior, settlement patterns, livelihoods, and socio-cultural activities. The following sub-chapters will elaborate in more depth the vulnerability of indigenous peoples.

3.1 Cognitive Aspects of Vulnerability: Indigenous Peoples' Perceptions Toward COVID-19

Cognitive elements has been widely used to determine subjective vulnerability. Canon (2015) emphasized that one's perception will decide whether or not he or she is vulnerable. According to his works, the perception toward environment and housing conditions, for instance, varies greatly from person to person. The majority of individuals who live in a disaster-prone area, for example, have found some sort of peace with their situation and believe that they are not in danger zones. However, for others, living in a danger area is risky and should be avoided. Subjective evaluations of a phenomenon will determine the levels of confidence in the surrounding conditions, which in turn will bring about certain capacities.

Perception is an internal mechanism that enables an individual to select, organize, and interpret stimuli from the surroundings, the process of which exerts an influence over his or her condition. Some scholars have identified numerous aspects that affects an individual's perception. Krech et al. (1962) also asserted that the following factors shape a person's perception: the first is a frame of reference, i.e., a body of knowledge influenced by education, reading materials, and studies; and the second is a frame of experience, i.e., events that have been encountered and are inseparable from the surrounding environments. Robbins (2003) added a number of factors that influence a person's perception. The first is attention, in which the focus is attended only to one or two objects rather than capturing all the surrounding stimuli at once. Different points of attention will lead to different perception. The second is person's mental preparation for the forthcoming stimuli. The third is individual's temporary or permanent needs by which his or her perception is determined. Different needs will result in different perceptions in each individual. The fourth is a value system adopted by a given society. The fifth is types of personality that will produce different perceptions in each individual.

Undoubtedly, a person's perception and understanding of the COVID-19 pandemic will influence the reaction to be taken. Someone will evaluate the presence of COVID-19 based on his or her perception of the situations. The evaluation will differ according to attitudes, knowledge, skills, and past experiences (Vibriyanti, 2020). An anxiety response will occur when the stressor is deemed harmful. On the other hand, abandonment will happen when the stressor is rendered non-threatening.

The research findings about the indigenous peoples' perceptions of COVID-19 are intriguing. People's perceptions of a phenomenon are influenced by knowledge, experiences, and cultures they believe in. When it comes to knowledge, this research found that that the peoples lacks sufficient information about COVID-19. A lot of information they obtain through social media failed to provide them with comprehensive and easy-to-understand explanations, causing uncertainty regarding the high risks of the pandemic. Their past experiences, particularly in coping with disease outbreaks like a pandemic, have given them a sort of strategic preparedness to deal with a plague or a pandemic.

Meanwhile, local culture has the greatest impact on how they perceive the pandemic and accordingly respond to it. In almost all the research sites, indigenous peoples rely heavily on their leaders for guidance and orders. When the rule prohibits them leaving the area, they will comply. This demonstrates that obedience to indigenous leaders remains the most important factor event though there are some differences in certain regions. For example, in Bali, which is a somewhat open or non-isolated region, they welcome a large number of returning migrants who left the village for years working in other towns outside the Islands of Bali. An open-armed attitude of the local people is one of the characteristics that makes it easier for the migrants to return to and begin a new life in the villages, particularly engaging in economic activities in agriculture and plantations for survival in the middle of the pandemic.

In general, nearly all areas exhibit a similar trend. Most of indigenous peoples do not perceive the epidemic as a significant threat to their life, but rather as a challenge that can be overcome. They seem to share almost the same perception although some individuals express their concerns about coping with this epidemic. For example, during a focus group discussion with the Marapu people of Sumba, one informant, who was also a survivor, felt very worried about COVID-19 due to a terrifying experience of being tested positive for the virus. Nevertheless, the majority of people do not take it as a serious threat to their lives. One explanation is because their past experiences revealed patterns of a similar disease in their residential areas, and all of them could be handled with traditional medicine practices and techniques unique to each indigenous group.

Knowledge-influenced perceptions of COVID-19 are also quite interesting to discuss in detail. Due to the current free flows of information through social media, everyone has unfettered access to information, which has led to the spread of irresponsible hoaxes. The findings in Bali and Sumba indicate that there is concern about visiting a health service facility for fear of being intentionally diagnosed with COVID-19 (*dikovidkan*). It is even more extreme that some of the Marapu people in Sumba believe that who goes to the hospital will certainly die. As a result, people prefer to remain at home and stick to the strategies they have used in dealing with the pandemics in the past. Meanwhile, the Nuaulu people have been aware that they are now facing the pandemic crisis and that the COVID-19 virus is real. They obtain information and news regarding the COVID-19 pandemic from a variety of electronic and social media that have become an integral part of their everyday life. The Nuaulu people is not a primitive, isolated tribe at this time.

This demonstrates that indigenous peoples had limited understanding of the COVID-19 pandemic. COVID-19-related knowledge is still limited to materials describing the condition of a rapidly spreading disease with various effects. The people know a little, particularly through reliable sources of information, about the consequences of the virus's spread. In addition to the limited knowledge, facts that the people witness and experience also shape how they perceive the COVID-19 pandemic. For example, the field works revealed that the public believes the COVID-19 mortality rate to be negligible in comparison to the cure rates of COVID-19 patients. This impacts how they respond to and prepare for the pandemic.

Some informants of the Nuaulu people claimed to have known the dangers of COVID-19 and the health protocols socialized by the government. However, they do not fully materialize this knowledge and understanding into behavioral changes. It can be said that wearing a mask, as one of the most efficient measures to prevent the spread of the virus, is limited to formal and official events, such as welcoming guests at the Saniri Office (Indigenous Government Office). In contrast, the Nuaulu indigenous people does not strictly follow health protocols such as wearing masks, maintaining distance, and washing hands in their daily lives. This is evident from the fact that traditional activities or rituals—such as the *Pinamou* (a rite of passage for adolescent into adulthood for women), the *Pataheri* (an initiation ritual for boys entering adulthood), and various dances, such as *maku-maku, cakalele*, and others—continue to be regularly held by the Nuaulu people, despite the pandemic.

Some of them believe that the symptoms caused by the COVID-19 virus only resemble "*batuk baringos*" or seasonal respiratory ailments. Mask-wearing is also very rare among the Nuaulu indigenous people. They argued that wearing a mask makes it difficult to breathe, and they believe that their living environment is safe from the threat of COVID-19. This sense of alleged safety comes from their very low mobility outside the village. They used to garden and hunt in the forest before returning to their houses. They leave the village just to be able to sell their plantation goods and hunt results in the city of Masohi.

In contrast to the Nuaulu people, the Balinese indigenous people are disciplined enough to wear masks. The indigenous villages, which are part of the COVID-19 task forces, have played a significant role in the implementation of disciplined health protocols. Unfortunately, discipline in wearing masks is not accompanied by strict adherence to health protocols when performing traditional activities such as rites of marriage, childbirth, and others. A crowd, no matter how small, remains potentially a place for the spread of COVID-19.

The field work found that the public's perception of the COVID-19 pandemic is low, which could put them in a vulnerable position. Nevertheless, the data also revealed that the indigenous peoples also have the capability or the potential to anticipate COVID-19 using their local knowledge, such as traditional healing systems and customary village rules, thus helping them become resilient in the face of the virus.

This is one of the capacities being materialized in accordance with local strategies and serves as an indicator of the low vulnerability of these indigenous groups.

In addition to looking at the perception of COVID-19 in relation to the level of vulnerability, it is also essential to examine the extent to which indigenous peoples are vulnerable in terms of their economic conditions. As is the case with the cognitive side of perception toward COVID-19, this study also scrutinizes how individuals perceive changes in their economic circumstances. In general, most people in nearly all the research sites feel that the COVID-19 pandemic does have an impact on their economies. One of them is the decline in tourist visits, which has a direct effect on all tourism-related industries. As a result, more workers are laid off, particularly in locations where tourism is the primary source of income, such as Bali and Sumba. From an economic standpoint, the perceptions of COVID-19 become intensified in which it is considered as an existential threat to them. But again, being faithful to what they have, i.e. daily traditional patterns or habits, they are not too perturbed about the economic impacts. Alternatively, they now turn to gardens or lands for cultivation, which they often used intermittently, as their main sources of livelihoods.

3.2 Age Group

According to a number of studies, the age factor contributes significantly to COVID-19 exposure levels and mortality rates (Oguz et al., 2021). This is because, for instance, the aged population and their concomitant diseases have an effect on the decline in their immune systems. A report by the World Health Organization (WHO) mentioned that more than 95% of COVID-19-related deaths occur in people older than 60 years of age. Moreover, according to statistics from the Task Force for the Acceleration of Handling COVID-19 of the Republic of Indonesia through May 2021 the elderly accounted for 49% of the COVID-19-related mortality rate. This fact demonstrates the significance of examining the vulnerability of indigenous peoples by age group.

Overall, the percentage of persons by age group at the research sites of indigenous peoples is dominated by the productive age group. Based on the SP2010 data, the percentage of the population over the age of 60 years does not exceed 10%. For instance, in Biak-Numfor District, approximately 9.7% of the people who are 60 years old or over. Sixty percent of the population of Biak-Numfor is comprised of productive-age individuals. As with the case of OAP in Biak-Numfor, the number of population aged 60 and older is relatively small, accounting for 8.5% of the Nuaulu indigenous people. Among the indigenous population of the Central Maluku District, children and adolescents account for 45.5% of the population. The percentage of the Orang Rimba population in Jambi who are 60 years of age or older is similarly less than 10%, or more precisely 5.4%. Roughly, 10% of the inhabitants of the Marapu village in East Nusa Tenggara is estimated to be over 60 years old. Among the residents who claimed to be the Tugutils, only one person is recorded in East Wasile, and 300 persons (164 men and 136 women) in North Maba. The majority of the Tugutils are comprised of youngsters (ages 5 to 9 years and 0 to 4 years), while the elderly people are very few.

However, one area of indigenous peoples has a rather high proportion of elderly residents, namely the Ngadas Village, where the Tengger indigenous people are dwelling. According to the population administration data from the Department of Population and Civil Registration of Malang District, 17.20% of the population in Ngadas Village is aged 0 to 14 years, 66.27% are 15 to 59 years old, and 16.53% are 60 years and over. Quantitatively, the percentage of eldery residents in Ngadas Village is lower than that of elderly people in Poncokusumo District and Malang District. Nevertheless, Ngadas Village has a relatively high percentage of elderly people, making them susceptible to COVID-19.

Meanwhile, the research in Bali found that the elderly population seem to be more vulnerable in general. This is evident from in-depth observations in the research location and interviews with local informants, who claimed that mortality due to COVID-19 was more prevalent among the older age group and the individuals with comorbidities. Nonetheless, it is important to note that the actual number of COVID-19 patients by age group is not possible to record due to the low number of tracings. Many individuals are reluctant to check themselves into health treatment centers and prefer instead self-isolation, for which reason they go unreported.

The fact that the indigenous population in the research site is dominated by productive age groups cannot be simplified as a low level of vulnerability among them. The reason is that, as mentioned earlier, vulnerability is complex and cannot be based on a single indicator. It is true that the younger age group is more resistant to the SarsCov-2 virus in this case, particularly when they have no history of disease or comorbidity. However, the largest percentage of young people in some areas of indigenous peoples can also put the elderly at risk. The younger-age population who engage in crowded activities, such as labor and trading, can potentially transmit the virus to the older people at home.

In addition to the age group of 60 years and above, the younger age group also deserves special attention during the pandemic. Adwiluvito and Rakhmawan (2020) found that children living in households wherein the heads of the families are working in the informal sector, having a low level of education, and are classified as poor will be more vulnerable to the effects of the COVID-19 pandemic. According to Kusumaningrum et al. (2021), the pandemic has increased the susceptibility of poor children, those with limited access to public services, and those who face discrimination based on their identification and social standing. Based on these findings, it is safe to conclude that the majority of indigenous peoples in the research sites are vulnerable. For instance, the Orang Rimba have a population composition of 46.3% children while the Nuaulu people 45.5% children of the total population. Even though they have received interventions from the government and NGOs, the conditions of the children in these two areas require additional attention during this pandemic, both in the form of educational and medical assistances.

3.3 Gender

The relationship between gender and the rate of COVID-19 infection has been extensively studied by scholars. Male gender is a risk factor for coronavirus infection (Susilo et al. 2020). In addition, these studies showed that the higher rate of active smokers among men is believed to be one of the contributing factors. This finding is also supported by other studies indicating that genetics, immunity, hormones, and masculine behavior or habits render men more susceptible to COVID-19 infection than women (Bwire, 2020; Capuano et al., 2020). However, a more recent research suggested that women are more susceptible to COVID-19 infection, but men continue to have the highest fatality rate (Kuehn, 2021). In light of these researches, what is the gender-specific vulnerability of indigenous populations to COVID-19?

In 2020, the total population of Biak-Numfor District was estimated to be 134,650, with 69,060 male and 65,560 female. Biak-Numfor District has a sex ratio of 105.29, which implies that for every 100 women, there are 105 men. In terms of gender, there were 1,519 cases of women tested positive for COVID-19 (55.56%). It has been hypothesized that the reason why COVID-19 affects more women than males is because women are more economically engaged in the market than men. The relatively high frequency of social interaction combined with improper application of health protocols increases the risk of virus transmission during business transactions. Many of them do not wear masks in the absence of government oversight. This is also related to the denial attitude and behavior to COVID-19. However, men are more likely to die from COVID-19 than women. A total of 79 man and 66 women were recorded to have died of coronavirus. Cigarette smoking habits are higher among males than females. Approximately 70% of men are smokers, according to the observations. This research found that there were patients who died with comorbidities triggered by smoking.

The Tenggerese people of Ngadas Village has a sex ratio of 107.7, which means that for every 100 female individuals, there are 107–108 male residents (BPS, 2021a). In other words, it has more male population than female. It is interesting to note that men and women work in the fields in the Tengger hamlet of Ngadas Village, hence they are equally at risk of getting infected with COVID-19. Smoking habits among the Tengger women have been underway since the days of their ancestors, therefore a smoking woman is a normal thing and is not contradictory with the applicable norms and standards among the Tenggerese people (Afifudin et al., 2018). Smoking cigarrete has become a habit in both men and women of the Tengger people in Ngadas Village. They like to smoke in the fields to repel coldness. One female informant said, "*Tiyang Tengger niki kalo mboten ngerokok anu, nek ting tenggil asrep.*"/ "*The Tenggerese People say that if they don't smoke, you know, up in the highlands they just feel cold.*" During pregnancy and breastfeeding, the Tengger women temporarily abstain from smoking before resuming the habit thereafter. But now the majority of women who are smoking are the elderly. The FGDs conducted in the research site found that women in a relatively young age group prefer not to smoke because they are aware of the dangers. However, the smoking habits among some Tengger people in Ngadas Village make people vulnerable to COVID-19 exposure.

Meanwhile, the SP 2010 data showed that the percentage of males and females within the Nuaulu indigenous people is almost identical: 50.5% males and 49.5% females. The Nuaulu is a patriarchal society in which most of men work outside their homes and most of women do all kinds of domestic affairs. Consequently, their household economies are heavily dependent on men. However, as times develop, women now have the same opportunities as men. Some of the Nuaulu women have earned bachelor's degrees, although their numbers are quite few.

The percentage of male and female within the Orang Rimba is almost equal: 1603 for men and 1602 for women. Similar to other regions, however, the Orang Rimba is also a patriarchal society. Therefore, men become the main buffers of household economies. The field research in Jambi found that the pandemic conditions made it extremely difficult for the family heads to meet their financial obligations. If the head of the household get infected with COVID-19, the rest of the family members will suffer even more. Despite the fact that the Orang Rimba have a strong sense of solidarity, in general they remain in uncertain and difficult conditions during the pandemic.

3.4 Population Mobility

Population mobility is one of the most essential indicators of vulnerability. First, someone with mobility has the potential to spread or contract the virus in the destination area. An upward and uncontrollable trend in population mobility is related to re-immigration of people who work outside of town but, due to loss of employment, have to return to their villages or region of origin.

The returning migrants can be divided into two groups: those who still own lands (either their own or that of their parents) and those who do not. The first group has an easier time adjusting to the place of origin and can be classified as a group that is less susceptible to the pandemic's effects, particularly when they suffered an immediate impact of losing their jobs. The second group consists of those who experience a major impact since, in addition to unemployment, they lack the financial resources to return to work in their home of origins. The second group falls within the category of economically vulnerable groups.

The trend to return to the village is noticeable in numerous research locations in Bali. The return of migrants who worked in centers of tourism activities happens almost thoroughly in all the areas. For them, returning to the village is a final resort due to the absence of other alternatives in urban regions. This remigration increases the vulnerability of both the migrant returnees and the host communities. Besides the spread of COVID-19, the availability of jobs or survival-related activities also becomes a serious concern.

Traveling by land transportation from their home village to Masohi City is a common pattern of mobility among the Nuaulu indigenous people. Due to the utilization of land, sea, and air transportation, the Nuaulu people become more susceptible to the spread of COVID-19 during the pandemic. This is because they come into contact with the outsiders from the Seram Island who may be positive for COVID-19 without symptoms (OTG). However, the local government has restricted the mobility of the Nuaulu people by reduction in the frequency of sea and air crossings; for example, during a pandemic sea crossings have been limited from twice per day to one per day. A Nuaulu informant from Tamilouw Village said that the Nuaulu people have preferred to postpone their working and school activities in Ambon City.

The Orang Rimba exhibit the same pattern of mobility, as they must move from one location to another for various reasons. According to the results of 2010 Population Census, migrations happened throughout the year in all six Orang Rimba-populated districts (Merangin, Sarolangun, Batang Hari, Tanjung Jabung Barat, Tebo, and Bungo). The highest in-migration was approximately 965 people in Tanjung Jabung Barat, while the lowest was 63 people in Batang Hari. Out-migration was highest in Batang Hari, with roughly 5418 individuals, and lowest in Tanjung Jabung Barat, with zero individuals (no out-migration).

In relation to migration, the Orang Rimba people has a unique or distinctive tradition called *belangun/melangun*, which is typically performed when a sorrowful event (death of a family member) happened in an Orang Rimba household. This migration activity is transient (also known as nonpermanent migration). The migration can last for two years, one year, six months, or only a few months or weeks. Certainly, this tradition can give a theoretical contribution to the existing concept or definition of migration.

The findings of research conducted in Ngadas Village showed that population stability and migration patterns are interrelated. According to several interviews with the Tenggerese people, population movement (in-migration and out-migration) in Ngadas Village occurred for several reasons. The first is employment for those assigned by their offices to work in Ngadas Village as teachers, health workers, and agricultural extension employees; the second is marriage for the villagers who married people from other areas and then settled in Ngadas Village or vice versa; the third is education for some inhabitants who had to go out of town for pursuing a higher education because educational facilities in Ngadas Village only extend to junior high school levels; and the fourth is economy for a small number of residents who chose to search for work and look for new experiences outside of the village. There are also residents who became Indonesian migrant workers, albeit in small numbers. It is interesting to note that the marriage system among the Tengger people has its own idiosyncrasies, which include its own noble values, and also influences migration trends. The marriage system among the Tengger society is both exogamous and heterogamous, meaning that there is no bar against marrying members of the community from different social strata or from outside the Tengger's indigenous people (Kurniawati et al., 2012; in Laksono, 2020). In carrying out their wedding processions, however, the Tenggerese women who marry men from other regions or outside the Tengger community must adhere to Tengger traditions and remain in the

Tengger region. Due to the importance of retaining land ownership, the majority of Tenggerese chose to marry fellow members of their own ethnic group.

The mobility pattern of the Tengger people in Ngadas Village is mostly driven by economic factors. They sell their agricultural products to the nearest market, collectors, or buyers who come to purchase their agricultural items. Tourism is the source of the subsequent mobility; the villagers rent jeeps or horses for crater excursions or homestays for tourists. In addition, educational considerations contribute to the everyday movement of rural communities; because the present educational facilities are only at the junior high school level, some inhabitants must go down (to the capital district of Poncokusumo) if they wish to complete their high school education. On the basis of the mobility factors of the outgoing population, it can be argued that the Tengger people of Ngadas Village are not susceptible to COVID-19 exposure due to their low population mobility.

3.5 Livelihood/Economy

One of the determinants of population vulnerability is livelihood. In this study, vulnerability is measured by susceptibility to COVID-19 and the impacts of its pandemic. It is quite often that a person's source of income is one of the primary markers that indicate his or her vulnerability. Tourism jobs, for instance, are the most fragile during this pandemic since they are one of the sectors that is directly affected by it. In addition, works connected to health services and those require a person to remain in a crowd and interact with a large number of people are classified as jobs that place an individual in a vulnerable position for COVID-19 transmission.

In general, this study identifies at least three major types of livelihoods, namely tourism, agriculture and plantations, and fisheries. People whose only source of income is tourism are the most susceptible compared to those who depend on agriculture or fisheries. When it comes to the transmission of COVID-19, however, the adherence of each individual to health protocols is a crucial aspect.

Bali is the only province in Indonesia to have seen the most severe effects of the pandemic. The fall in economic growth reached −12 and lasted for a considerable amount of time. This indicates that there are a significant number of individuals in the tourism industry that must be laid off, while some can continue to work part time. The indirect secondary effect is that a massive deal of economic activity that supports tourism become eventually inflicted. Tourism-related economic activities include drivers, souvenir sellers, food vendors, and workers in various service sectors. As soon as the pandemic struck, all workers in numerous fields were immediately hampered. Regarding their susceptibility to COVID-19 transmission, workers in Bali's tourism industry are notably less visible because all tourism-related activities have ceased to operate. However, when the tourism industry reopens for a while, particularly for domestic tourists, tourism employees are the most vulnerable and first to be hit. As was the case in Indonesia in general, the holiday season in July 2021 was a time when tourism workers undergo a very high degree of transmission phase. Due to the spread of a highly contagious and lethal delta variant of COVID-19, workers become the most vulnerable to the effects of the coronavirus disease.

After returning to their villages and resuming economic activities, however, the workers' vulnerability has changed. The majority of them continued to farming and plantation works once they had moved to their places of origin, which made them less vulnerable to COVID-19 because their activities were predominantly conducted in the outdoors. Nevertheless, back to their socio-cultural activities, they are attracted to large crowds again. When a large group of people participate in traditional rituals, there is a chance for the virus to spread and be transmitted.

The Nuaulu indigenous people have unique ways of livelihoods. Living and residing along the seaside does not necessarily give the locals proficiency at fishing. Despite living near the shore, the bulk of the Nuaulu people is comprised of gardeners and horticulturists who cultivate cassava, corn, coconut, cloves, cocoa, vegetables, and fruits. This is tightly related to the fact that the Nuaulu people are typologically mountain-dwellers less familiar with marine culture (Kristiansen et al., 2021). In addition, the Nuaulu people make a living through rearing livestock (chickens and cows), working as government officials, particularly in the hamlet or village office, and trading. One explanation for this condition is that their forefathers lived in the hills or mountains and knew little about marine life, thereby making it nearly impossible for them to become fisherman. A tiny portion of the Nuaulu population are indeed adept at catching fish in the sea, but they learned this skill from their experience working with the Bugis and Butonese who live there. The Nuaulu people, particularly those who live close to the coast (Rounusa Hemlet, Sepa Village), have a strong desire to be able to fish in the ocean, but they are unable to do so due to a lack of fishing facilities and infrastructure such as boats, propulsion engines, nets, fishing equipment, as well as capital. They inevitably rely on selling their agricultural and plantation products to other regions, especially Masohi City, because they only possess farming and gardening abilities. Their low marketability makes them dependent on agricultural product collectors from Masohi City, whose operations during the pandemic were restricted due to social distancing policies. This produces a significant decline in their revenue.

The agriculture sector accounts for 90% of the Tengger's primary source of income in Ngadas Village, which is the highest proportion among the major economic activities. This contrasts with Malang District, where 43.91% of the workforce is employed in the service industry (BPS, 2021b). Agriculture is the main livelihood for the Tengger's people of Ngadas, the majority of whom are field farmers (in the southern villages); some also rear cattle and work as laborers and grass seekers. Ngadas Village is situated within the boundaries of Bromo Tengger Semeru National Park (TNBTS). Thus, Ngadas Village also becomes a tourist attraction and destination and tourism serves as an extra source of income. On average, they are jeep owners, jeep rental service providers, homestays owners, small traders (meatballs, coffee, t-shirts, etc.), and brokers (*keber*). As a result of the COVID-19 pandemic and the imposition of community activity restrictions (PPKM), the Bromo tourist area was closed to visitors, and those who worked in the tourism industry were forced to find new employment. The residents of Ngadas returned to their primary occupation, which is in agriculture. Our observations indicated that the farmers operate in a rather large enough land, thereby allowing them to maintain social distance. When working in the fields, the farmers receive adequate air circulation and sunlight. In this regard, the Tengger's residents of Ngadas Village are typically less susceptible to COVID-19.

Other indigenous peoples were also confronted with economic challenges even before the pandemic. For example, the Orang Rimba suffer even more in the midst of the COVID-19 pandemic, which has compelled them to make certain adjustments. They are socially and economically vulnerable. As described in the preceding section, the Orang Rimba have limited access to health, education, and economic facilities. Even if the Orang Rimba have gotten considerable attention in recent years from the regional and central governments as well as civil society organizations, the pandemic condition makes the adaptation process more challenging. The Orang Rimba are becoming increasingly vulnerable as their living space is getting narrower. Nevertheless, the Orang Rimba who cultivate gardens in the forest are generally unaffected economically although commodity prices have decreased, especially for red-resin (jernang), dammar, and rattan.

The OAP of Biak-Numfor also shows economic vulnerability due to the COVID-19 pandemic. Compared to the past, things have changed significantly in the present. In the past, the people of Biak-Numfor used to rely on fishing, sago harvesting, and hunting as their primary source of income. Along with the presence of the government and the church, the urban-dwelling Papuans serve in the government bureaucracy, both civil and military, as teachers, medical professionals, pastors, and in the commercial sectors as sellers of areca nut, knotted woven bag (*noken*), and fisheries or agricultural products. The Papuans residing in rural or coastal areas are mostly farmers, copra producers, and fisherman. The coming of several ethnic groups from outside Biak-Numfor, both Papuans and non-Papuans, have fostered the growth of employment prospects in the private sector, including hotels, restaurants, transportation, banking, and fish processing, which may be hampered because of the pandemic. Unfortunately, the industrial sector in this region has not yet developed and has been limited to small enterprises of copra, coffee, and wood processing.

3.6 Health Behaviors

Health behaviors are one of the indicators that determine whether a person vulnerable or not. In this study, there are two categories of health behaviors. The first is daily activities that reflect traditions and cultures that a community preserves in everyday life. The second is health behaviors linked to the directives and policies given by both the central and local governments.

The Nuaulu indigenous peoples have an excellent knowledge of herbs. They are familiar with numerous leaves, plants, and even fruits that can be used to treat various ailments. They usually use some type of leaves for medicine, such as those of star fruit (*belimbing*) for high blood pressure, jatropha (*pohon jarak*) for heat illness, *daun biana* for ulcers, itchy leaves for fatigue, and the roots of the weeds for malaria, and *daun bentang* for fever. In addition to using traditional medicines, some of them have begun to seek medical care at the local public health centers (*Puskesmas*). They are willing to receive further treatment and healing if traditional medicine fails to give positive results. According to the focus group discussion, they continue to believe in their ancestral teachings on health. Furthermore, they gain knowledge about health through contacts with individuals outside of their community as well as via television, social media, and the internet.

The Survey on People's Behaviors amid the COVID-19 Pandemic conducted by the BPS in 13–20 July 2021 showed that the degree of community compliance with health protocols is relatively high, particularly in Java-Bali (BPS, 2021c). Nevertheless, according to our observation in Ngadas Village, the Tenggerese are still rarely seen wearing masks in daily life, except when they were invited to the meetings or FGDs. It is uncommon to find a hand-washing station or hand sanitizer on the terrace of their residences. The tradition of "*Apen-apen,*" in which neighbors congregate in close proximity to a fire to warm their bodies while chatting, also still occurs. During the pandemic, traditional rites involving crowds such as the *Walagara* ceremony (traditional wedding), are still held, albeit with restrictions on the number of participants and adherence to health protocols like wearing masks. It can be argued that this crowd behavior has put the Ngadas peoples at higher risk of contracting COVID-19. However, it is important to note that this behavior was also the result of negotiation between customs (*adat*) on the one side and the COVID-19 government regulations on the other.

The ease with which people can obtain medical care also influences their public health behaviors. Due to their location in the center of the village and the limited mobility of health workers, the forest-dwelling Tugutil continue to have difficulty accessing health facilities such as physicians, midwives, community health centers (*puskesmas*) and community health sub-centers (*puskesmas pembantu*). When there are serious health issues, such as difficult births, severe injuries, and chronic diseases, it will be difficult for them to receive immediate assistance. Meanwhile, the village-dwelling Tugutil people have easier access to medical facilities. The Tugutil people living in the forests and in the villages are also susceptible to a variety of other ailments, including skin diseases and diarrhea, because of inadequate sanitation. Due to their reliance on river water for sanitation, the forest-dwelling Tugutil people prefer to defecate in the forest rather than the river. In addition, the government housing program dwellings built in Titipa Hamlet and Tukur-Tukur Hamlet did not provide toilets in each house; instead, only community toilets were installed, which were subsequently abandoned. The rationale is that sanitation in a community is more individual than collective.

3.7 Settlement Pattern

One of the criteria for identifying the vulnerability of indigenous peoples is the pattern of settlement. Clustered settlements are prevalent among indigenous peoples but nomadic ones are still noticeable in some of them although in very small numbers. However, communality and kinship are quite strong among indigenous peoples. Based on the findings at the research site, many indigenous peoples who live in clustered dwellings, particularly in urban areas, such as the Nuaulu, the Bali Aga, and the OAP, have integrated with society as a whole. This condition may result in different degrees of vulnerability among indigenous peoples.

The research conducted within the Nuaulu Tribe found that their settlements are typically located in the highlands with some distance from the coast. The Nuaulu Tribe builds houses or dwellings on the land in accordance with their respective customary lands that already exist in residential areas. The dwelling structures of the Nuaulu people are typically constructed adjacent to country roads or villages. Some houses are on stilts, while others are on the ground. Some traditional dwellings of the Nuaulu Tribe still use sago leaf or sago pelepa (*gaba-gaba*) for roofs, plank and bamboo for walls (stilt houses), or dirt for floors (landed houses). Other dwellings, however, are similar to decent houses in general, with timber pillars or clapboard walls, zinc roofs, and cement flooring. Some houses are even constructed with tiled flooring and modern architectural shapes.

Although the Decree of the Minister of Health of the Republic of Indonesia Number HK.01.07/MENKES/413/2020 about Guidelines for the Prevention and Control of Coronavirus Disease 2019 (COVID-19) mentions that COVID-19 can be prevented by routinely washing hands with soap and water, during the pandemic not a single house in the Nuaulu Tribe provided a soap-hand washing station for visitors or guests. However, the Nuaulu people have their own health protocol mechanisms.

In contrast to the Nuaulu people, who have been affected by modernization, the forest-dwelling Tugutils often lead a semi-nomadic lifestyle and are dispersed in hard-to-reach locations. The food supplies in the forest contribute to this nomadic way of living. The forest-dwelling Tugutil people are not registered in the population administration due to their locations that are scattered and far away from the governance centers, let alone their reading and writing illiteracy. Most of the Tugutil people are not recorded in the population administration system, making it impossible to gather data on their number and whereabouts. Moreover, the forest-dwelling Tugutils can have multiple names for the same individual, making double registration more likely. The fact that most Tugutil people are unregistered in the population administration system has caused delays in the delivery of health and education services.

3.8 Socio-Cultural Activities

Socio-economic dynamics in relation to catastrophes (including a social disaster of pandemic) cannot be separated from customs, beliefs, and habits that people continue to preserve in daily life (Krüger et al., 2015). One obstacle in slowing down the spread of pandemic cases has been crowds stir up by traditional festivals or other practices that involve a large number of individuals in a particular residential area. According to numerous news reports, traditional ceremonies have become one of the clusters responsible for the rapid spread of the virus.

The Nuaulu tribe is renowned for the preservation of their indigenous culture. Based on our observations and interviews, the Nuaulu people do not exhibit any changes in behaviors during the pandemic, particularly in their ritual and cultural activities. They continues to conduct all stages of traditional and religious rites. They believe the COVID-19 virus does not really exist in their community, hence there is no reason to refrain from performing traditional and religious festivals. This is evident from the research team's observations of a ceremony that involves sending a girl to the *posune (seclusion house)*. The women were cooking as usual, with no one wearing a mask or maintaining a physical distance. The same case is true when we attended the *Maku-Maku* traditional ceremony in Ronnusa hamlet, wherein the participants are dancing together in a circular form holding each other all night. The performance began at 21.00 and concluded when the sun rises the next morning. No COVID-19 health protocol was implemented during the *Maku-Maku* dance ceremony. Even the habit of chewing betel nut and spitting out the residual was still prevalent at the event. In the context of the their susceptibility to the spread of COVID-19, it can be claimed that the Nuaulu people are a vulnerable group, since their persistence in performing traditional and religious activities during the pandemic has opened a loophole that requires attention in relation to the virus transmission.

For the Tengger people, traditional rites are an integral part of their daily life and are a manifestation of their continued existence as a group that still holds firm their local customs. The Tengger people of Ngadas Village are a community that adheres to and practices their own traditions and rituals relying on the Spirit of the Mountain for protection. Changes in socio-economic, cultural, and religious landscapes in the region did not dampen their passion for traditional rituals and festivities. For them, traditional rites are synonymous with the many values to which they adhere, and they always carry out customs in accordance with their religious and ancestral beliefs. The frequency and amplitude of the customary rites that the Tengger people of Ngadas Village must perform have the potential to contribute to the spread of COVID-19. It is believed that community participation in big numbers and crowds can expedite the transmission of the COVID-19 virus. Therefore, customs and traditions alone can be a vulnerability factor in Ngadas Village. The co-celebration of religious holidays and traditional rites, which have evolved into Tenggerese traditions and customs, is an additional risk factor for COVID-19 exposure. Thousands of people always attend every *Kasada* event, for instance.

Similar to the people of Central Maluku and the Tengger Tribe, the lives of indigenous people in Bali is inextricably linked to traditional practices. The distinctiveness in performing traditional rites is the most intriguing aspect of the studied community groups as compared to other Balinese in general. The indigenous people being studied were the Bali Aga and Bali Mula, i.e. communities who claimed to have existed prior to the influence of the Javanese Majapahit Kingdom. More specifically, the traditional rites being performed are founded on their belief in the nobility of Water, for which reason they call themselves as believers of "*Piagem Game Tirte*" or a religion that is wholly dependent on the existence of a water source, which in this case is Tamblingan Lake.

In order to control the spread of COVID-19 in Bali, restrictions on activities, including traditional ones, are imposed. The Governor of Bali issued a Circular Letter No. 07 of 2021 on the extension of village/urban commune-based PPKM, which is then accompanied by the Parisada Hindu Dharma (PHDI) Circular Letter No. 076/ PHDI Bali/VIII/2021 regulating the types of rituals that could be performed by the Balinese Hindu communities. When the PPKM level 4 is implemented, the number of participants in traditional rituals, such as funerals and weddings, is restricted to no more than ten individuals. It is also advised that each family's place of worship be used for activities that would be normally carried out in groups.

In conjunction with the extension of Level 4 Community Activity Restrictions (PPKM) in Java and Bali, Parisadha Hindu Dharma Indonesia (PHDI) Bali and the Traditional Village Council (MDA) of Bali Province published a Circular Letter (SE) concerning restrictions on traditional rites. The circular letters of No. 076/ PHDI-Bali/VIII/2021 and No. 008/SE/MDA-Prov. Bali/VIII/2021 govern all types of ceremonies in *Panca.*

An interesting aspect to note is the distinctiveness with which the people of Bali Aga or Bali Mula observe their traditions and rituals, particularly with regard to death ceremonies or *Ngaben.* The ritual of cremation or the burning of bodies, the timing of which is determined by a number of factors, is the final ceremonial for the majority of Bali's residents. In contrast, for the Bali Aga people, the procession of death is carried out not through the *Ngaben* ceremony, but through burial.

It is obvious that death ceremonies could attract a large crowd. A modest procession, however, can lessen the likelihood of crowds and the intensity of physical and social interactions. In addition to the death procession, there is also difference between the Bali Aga and the average Balinese people in routinely holding religious ceremonies according to the Balinese calendar. The performance of religious rites by the Bali Aga people is less intense because all religious activities are consolidated every two years into one huge main event. The biannual traditional ceremonies have also a profound significance for nature conservation and social harmony.

During the pandemic, traditional ceremonies are also still held in Biak-Numfor. The belief system of Biak indigenous people is fundamentally comparable to those of other indigenous communities in the Land of Papua or the Archipelago. They believe in a supernatural force known as "*fan nanggi*" and refer to the God who rules the universe as "*manseren nanggi.*" Various rituals or cultural practices in the past have always been associated with reverence and belief in ancestor spirits, who are believed to potentially bring bad consequences for the community, such as war and natural disasters. In the past, diverse transitional ceremonies included stepping foot on earth (*sababu*), initiation (*k'bor*), and hair cutting (*kapanakzik*). However, these traditional ceremonies have been superseded by church rituals such as baptism and confirmation of faith.

Bali: Lessons from the COVID-19 Pandemic for Economic Transformation

Bali is one of the areas studied to determine how indigenous peoples and the effects of the pandemic correlate with the socio-demographical conditions. Bali becomes an interesting area of study to explore the tremendous economic impacts experienced by the community as a result of the tourism sector's dominance in supporting the local economy. Meanwhile, the focus of the study in Bali is on indigenous peoples with distinctive traditions and beliefs compared to the Balinese population in general. The indigenous peoples of "Bali Aga" and "Bali Mula" in Banjar Sub-District, Buleleng District, are the subjects of this study.

This study employs two concepts of vulnerability when examining the susceptibility of indigenous peoples to the pandemics in Bali: the first is based on cognitive measurements and the second on measurable quantitative indicators.

Economic Transformation in Bali: Lessons from the COVID-19 Pandemic

As mentioned in the preceding section, the paralysis of tourism industry has also crippled the economy in Bali. Due to the shutdown of domestic and international travel tourism, many hotels and inns had to lay off their personnel. As a result, other supporting industries, including services and commerce, suffer a sharp reduction in activity. The increasing number of layoffs, wage cuts, and temporary layoffs has also elevated the unemployment rate in Bali.

During 2019–2020, the number and rate of unemployment increased dramatically, resulting in a rise in the number of individuals living in poverty. Although the percentage of poor individuals in rural areas is higher than in urban areas, the poverty rate in urban areas has increased significantly more than in rural ones (see Table 3.1).

When it comes to cities and districts, Buleleng District is one of the districts where the percentage of poor people has increased, along with Denpasar City. In

Table 3.1 Percentage of poor population in Bali Province

Area classification	Poor population in Bali province by area classification (percentage)					
	March			September		
	2019	2020	2021	2019	2020	2021
Urban Areas	3.29	3.33	4.12	3.04	4.04	–
Rural Areas	4.88	4.78	5.52	4.86	5.40	–
Urban + Rural Areas	3.79	3.78	4.53	3.61	4.45	–

Since 20,211 the provincial poverty rate was released twice a year, i.e. March and September period. Source: National Socio-Economic Survey

Source BPS (2021d)

Table 3.2 Average expenditure per capita by district/city in Bali

District/city	Average expenditure per capita by district/city in Bali (Thousand Rupiah)		
	2018	2019	2020
Jembrana District	11,666	11,902	11,790
Tabanan District	14,245	14,608	14,494
Badung District	17,325	17,628	17,503
Gianyar District	14,376	14,023	14,544
Klungkung District	11,318	11,484	11,376
Bangli District	11,160	11,369	11,268
Karangasem District	11,050	10,302	10,237
Buleleng District	13,235	13,780	13,463
Denpasar City	19,098	19,992	19,723
Bali Province	13,886	14,146	13,929

Source BPS (2021e)

2020, 5.32% of the population was poor, up from 5.19% in 2019, which represented a drop compared to the condition in 2018, which is 5.36%.

The increase in poverty is also mirrored by a decline in consumption or average per capita expenditure. When comparison is made between 2019 and 2020, Buleleng District suffered a drop (see Table 3.2),

The impact of the pandemic on the social system, the people, and the living system in general will determine the responses and strategies for dealing with the pandemic. The strategies being carried out can be seen from several levels, ranging from the government as a whole to the public. Ideally, the techniques used at all levels should be consistent and mutually supportive. The government's strategies should provide chances and room for local capacity-building initiatives.

The fragility of Bali's tourism industry has begun to be felt not only since the start of the pandemic in 2020, when people's mobility across regional borders was entirely restricted. Far beforehand, the acts of terrorism (the Bali Bombings in 2002 and 2005) and the disastrous eruption of Mount Agung in 2017 had slowed down the tourism industry in Bali. A discourse has developed afterward among some Balinese, particularly the youth, who believe that the tourism industry is no longer significant enough to serve as Bali's sole economic pillar. Subsequently, agriculture is one of the most prominent options recommended to reduce Bali's reliance on the tourism industry. In this context, "Tourism is a Bonus" becomes one of the taglines continuously amplified to the point where tourism is only viewed as an effect. In the meantime, the agricultural sector must be developed to become Bali's primary economic base. However, it is worth noting that the development of the agricultural sector has inherently spiritual significance for the Balinese people in addition to its economic worth.

The COVID-19 pandemic, which has been ongoing since 2020, has become a significant momentum in showing that the agricultural sector in Bali survived pretty well while the tourism sector was at its lowest point. Many people who formerly relied on tourism activities in the hubs of Bali's tourism industry have lost their jobs and have returned to their home villages. Gobleg Village and Munduk Village, situated in the customary village areas of Tamblingan of Buleleng District, were two of the villages where many tourism players returned to their home villages. According to the Office Head of Banjar Asah Gobleg, at least 200 family heads, the majority of them had previously worked in the tourism industry, returned to the village. Some of them then decided to work on either family-owned or rented agricultural lands.

Banjar Asah Gobleg is one of the areas in Buleleng District that has been long growing as an agricultural center. In the 1980s, coffee farming attracted people to move into this otherwise forested region. Many residents of Banjar Asah Gobleg began to replace their coffee plants with blue flowers and oranges at times when the coffee commodity was no longer seen as a guarantee of their well-being. Blue flowers and oranges eventually became the two primary crops grown by the majority of the inhabitants. Meanwhile, horticultural crops were later flourished by a young group known as the Keren Gobleg Young Farmers organization, or hereinafter abbreviated as PMK Gobleg. Banjar Asah Gobleg, which is topographically characterized by flat terrain, has the potential to become an agricultural hub when the bulk of land in Desa Adat Dalam Tamblingan, later abbreviated as DADT, is dominated by perennials, with cloves being the primary commodity.

The regeneration of farmers in all areas, including DADT, has stalled since the advent of the tourism industry in Bali. Many then choose to work in the tourism hubs in urban places outside of their villages. Many rice fields in Munduk Village, for instance, have been converted into clove plantations because there are no longer young people wanting to continue their parents' works in the fields. The majority of the seasonal labor (clove pickers) in the clove gardens in Munduk Village comes from outside the area. In Banjar Asah Gobleg, many family-owned lands have been abandoned because some of their youth view tourism as a more promising path to prosperity than farming; at least this was the case until the emergence of the PMK Gobleg that initiated a community-based agricultural movement and the implementation of digital technology with horticultural plants as their primary commodity.

The PMK Gobleg was established in 2019 by a group of young villagers who desired to boost the agricultural sector in their community. Since 2015, this organization has emerged as a farmer movement that seeks the growth of the agricultural industry. This organization began when a guy named Gede Suardita and other young people was joining the Bali Young Farmers Forum network founded by another young man named Agung Wedhatama. The objective is to encourage more young groups to return to the agricultural sector. Through a network with the Bali Young Farmers Forum, the PMK Gobleg aims to strengthen the rural agricultural sector from upstream to downstream, beginning with seed production, land preparation, planting, maintenance, harvesting, and selling. In fact, the term "young" is so fluid that the membership of PMK Gobleg, which consists of approximately 20 farmers, includes not only young farmers, but also people over the age of 50 who keep the spirit of becoming creative, innovative, and productive.

The PMK Gobleg is taking an increasingly growing role during the COVID-19 pandemic. The pandemic and the policy on people's mobility restrictions seemed to have no significant impact on the activities of the PMK Gobleg. However, there has been a drop in the demand for horticultural vegetable products during the pandemic. They anticipate this impact by managing cropping patterns that limit production quantities while expanding the varieties of vegetables planted and maintaining the sustainability of production.

References

Adwiluvito, H., & Rakhmawan, S.A. (2020). Proposing Additional Indicators Related to COVID-19 to the Children's Social Vulnerability Index in Indonesia. *International Conference on Data Analytics for Business and Industry: Way Towards a Sustainable Economy (ICDABI)*, Sakheer, 1–5. https://doi.org/10.1109/ICDABI51230.2020.9325694S

Adger, W.N. (2006). Vulnerability. *Global Environmental Change, 16*(3). 268–281. https://doi.org/10.1016/j.gloenvcha.2006.02.006

Afifudin, L., Dewi, F. S. T., & Padmawati, R. S. (2018) Budaya merokok wanita suku tengger. *Berita Kedokteran Masyarakat Journal of Community Medicine and Public Health, 34*(11), 403–410. https://doi.org/10.22146/bkm.36505

Bwire, G. M. (2020). Coronavirus: Why men are more vulnerable to COVID-19 than women? *SN Comprehensive Clinical Medicine, 2*(7), 874–876.

BPS (2021a). *Kecamatan Poncokusumo dalam Angka 2021.*

BPS (2021b). *Statistik Daerah Kabupaten Malang 2021.*

BPS (2021c). *Perilaku masyarakat pada masa PPKM darurat: Hasil survei perilaku masyarakat pada masa pandemi COVID-19 Periode 13-20 Juli 2021.*

BPS (2021d). Persentase Penduduk Miskin Provinsi Bali Menurut Klasifikasi Daerah (Persen) 2019–2021. *BPS Provinsi Bali.* https://bali.bps.go.id/id/statistics-table/2/NzAjMg==/persentase-penduduk-miskin-provinsi-bali-menurut-klasifikasi-daerah.html

BPS (2021e). Rata-rata Pengeluaran Per Kapita Disesuaikan Provinsi Bali Menurut Kabupaten/Kota (Ribu Rupiah) 2018–2020. *BPS Provinsi Bali.* https://bali.bps.go.id/id/statistics-table/2/NzAjMg==/persentase-penduduk-miskin-provinsi-bali-menurut-klasifikasi-daerah.htmlX

Bohle, H. G. (2001). Vulnerability and criticality: perspectives from social geography. *IHDP update, 2*(01), 3–5.

Canon, T. (2015). Disasters, Climate Change and the Significance of Culture. In F.Krüger., G. Bankoff, T. Cannon., B.Orlowski., & E.L.F. Schipper. *Culture and Disaster: Understanding Cultural Framings in Disaster Risk Reduction.* https://doi.org/10.4324/9781315797809

Capuano, A., Rossi, F., & Paolisso, G. (2020). COVID-19 kills more men than women: An overview of possible reasons. *Frontiers in Cardiovascular Medicine, 7*(131), 1–7. https://doi.org/10.3389/fcvm.2020.00131

Cardona, O. D., van Aalst, M. K., Birkmann, J., Fordham, M., McGregor, G., Perez, R., Pulwarty, R. S., Schipper, E. L. F., & Sinh, B. T. (2012). Determinants of risk: Exposure and vulnerability. In C. B. Field, V. Barros, T. F. Stocker, D. Qin, D. J. Dokken, K. L. Ebi, M. D. Mastrandrea, K. J. Mach, G.-K. Plattner, S. K. Allen, M. Tignor & P. M. Midgley (Eds.), *Managing the risks of extreme events and disasters to advance climate change adaptation. A special report of working groups I and II of the Intergovernmental Panel on Climate Change (IPCC)* (pp. 65–108). Cambridge University Press. https://www.ipcc.ch/site/assets/uploads/2018/03/SREX-Chap2_FINAL-1.pdf

Chambers, R. (1989). Editorial Introduction: Vulnerability, Coping and Policy. *IDS Bulletin, 20*(2), 1–7. https://doi.org/10.1111/j.1759-5436.1989.mp20002001.x
Dutta, I., Foster, J., & Mishra, A. (2011). On measuring vulnerability to poverty. *Social Choice and Welfare, 37*(4), 743–761. https://doi.org/10.1007/s00355-011-0570-1
Garschagen, M. (2014). *Risky change? Vulnerability and adaptation between climate change and transformation dynamics in Can Tho City, Vietnam*. Franz Steiner Verlag.
Krech, D., Crutchfield, R. S., & Ballachey, E. L. (1962). Individual in society: A textbook of social psychology. McGraw Hill Kogakhusa
Kristiansen, S., Budiman, A., & Pudyatmoko, S. (2021). Ecosystem guardians, or threats? Livelihood security and nature conservation in Maluku, Indonesia. *Bulletin of Indonesian Economic Studies*, 1–33. https://doi.org/10.1080/00074918.2021.1932744
Krüger, F., Bankoff, G., Cannon, T., Orlowski, B., & Schiper, L.F. (2015). *Cultures and Disasters: Understanding Cultural Framings in Disaster Risk Reduction*. Routledge. https://doi.org/10.4324/9781315797809
Kuehn, B. M. (2021). COVID-19 in Clinicians—more cases in women, more deaths in men. *JAMA, 325*(15), 1498–1498. https://doi.org/10.1001/jama.2021.5500
Kurniawati, P. I., Dinastiti, C., Ningtias, Y. K., Khoiriyah, S., & Putri, N. A. (2012). Potret Sistem Perkawinan Masyarakat Tengger di Tengah Modernitas Industri Pariwisata. https://doi.org/10.15294/solidarity.v1i1.215
Kusumaningrum, S., Siagian, C., & Beazley, H. (2021). Children during the COVID-19 pandemic: Children and young people's vulnerability and wellbeing in Indonesia. *Children's Geographies*, 1–11. https://doi.org/10.1080/14733285.2021.1900544
Laksono, A. D. (2020). Tengger bertahan dalam adat: studi konstruksi sosial ukuran keluarga suku Tengger. *Health Advocacy*.
Lancet, T. (2020). Redefining vulnerability in the era of COVID-19. *Lancet (London, England), 395*(10230), 1089. https://doi.org/10.1016/S0140-6736(20)30757-1
Niko, N. (2020). Poor and hunger: How do indigenous peoples' respond to COVID-19 in Indonesia? *Journal of Community Development Research (Humanities and Social Sciences), 14*(1), 81–92. https://doi.org/10.14456/jcdr-hs.2021.8
Oguz, S. H., Koca, M., & Yildiz, B. O. (2021). Aging versus youth: Endocrine aspects of vulnerability for COVID-19. *Reviews in Endocrine and Metabolic Disorders*, 1–20.https://doi.org/10.1007/s11154-021-09656-y
Power, T., Wilson, D., Best, O., Brockie, T., Bearskin, L. B., Millender, E., & Lowe, J. (2020). COVID-19 and indigenous peoples: An imperative for action. *Journal of Clinical Nursing*. https://doi.org/10.1111/jocn.15320
Robbins, S. P. (2003). *Organizational Behavior*. Upper Saddle River, NJ: Pearson Education.
Sen, A. K. (1981). *Poverty and famines: An essay on entitlement and deprivation*. Oxford.
Vibriyanti, D. (2020). Kesehatan mental masyarakat: mengelola kecemasan di tengah pandemi COVID-19. *Jurnal Kependudukan Indonesia*, 69–74. https://doi.org/10.14203/jki.v0i0.550
Wisner, B., Blaikie, P., Cannon, T., & Davis, I. (2004). *At risk: Natural hazards, people's vulnerability and disasters*. Routledge.

Chapter 4
The COVID-19 Pandemic and Its Impacts on Changes in Social and Demographic Conditions of Indigenous Peoples

Deshinta Vibriyanti, Triyono, Achsanah Hidayatina, Diah Ikawati, Uray Naviandi, Alfina Fasriani, and Al Huda Yusuf

Abstract This chapter illustrates the socio-demographic impacts of the COVID-19 pandemic on indigenous people in Indonesia, focusing on fertility, health and mortality, mobility, economy, and traditional rituals. Likewise, different measures set up by the government to address and manage the COVID-19 pandemic have unquestionably exerted influence over the community. Vibriyanti et al. explain that not all of the effects of the COVID-19 pandemic on the demographic aspect are directly visible in a short period of time. Looking at the statistical changes, the impacts of the COVID-19 pandemic on Indonesia's demographic condition will be most likely noticeable within one or two years. However, the nearly two-year-long COVID-19 pandemic has undoubtedly had a significant impact on the trend in demography-related behavioral changes that will shape the future demographic condition of a country, including Indonesia. The wave of the COVID-19 pandemic also has a negative effect on the socio-economic condition of the population. In this chapter, there are five sections that describe the effects of the COVID-19 pandemic on socio-demographic aspects of indigenous people, such as fertility, health and mortality rates, population mobility, economy, and traditional rituals. In general, COVID-19 has a minor impact on the mortality rates of indigenous populations. Indigenous people impacted by COVID-19, particularly in terms of population mobility, can be classified into two categories: those whose migration patterns remained unchanged,

D. Vibriyanti (✉) · Triyono
Research Center for Population, National Research and Innovation Agency (BRIN), Jakarta, Indonesia
e-mail: desh001@brin.go.id

A. Hidayatina
Research Center for Behavioral and Circular Economy, National Research and Innovation Agency (BRIN), Jakarta, Indonesia

D. Ikawati · U. Naviandi · A. Fasriani · A. H. Yusuf
Directorate of Population and Manpower Statistics, BPS-Statistics Indonesia, Jakarta, Indonesia

C. Pamungkas et al. (eds.), *The Impact of the Pandemic on Indigenous People in Indonesia*, Quality of Life in Asia 20, https://doi.org/10.1007/978-981-96-4222-9_4

and those whose mobility was disrupted by pandemic restrictions. The first is indigenous individuals whose migration habits and culture are not significantly impacted by the COVID-19 pandemic. The second group consists of indigenous individuals whose movement patterns have been altered by the COVID-19 pandemic. Moreover, the policies in regard to controlling the COVID-19 spread also have effects on population mobility. The decline of tourism severely reduced income for groups such as the Bali Aga, Marapu in Sumba, and the Tengger in East Java, whose cultural assets had become key economic commodities. The natural and cultural wealth owned by those indigenous peoples becomes a magnet for tourists to visit the regions. For instance, crafts such as woven fabrics, plaits, and traditional gold and silver jewelry, which had no commercial value to the Merapu people at first, have now become one of the community's economic commodities. However, the rules that restrict population mobility have rendered tourism completely inactive. The pandemic, which has been ongoing for almost two years, has had a substantial effect on the tourism industry. Furthermore, the portrayal of indigenous peoples' perspectives and understanding of the COVID-19 pandemic depicts how they live in the face of the threat posed by the virus's spread. The pandemic has had a minimal effect on the observance of cultural and religious practices. In this chapter, Vibriyanti et al. stated that the fear of COVID-19 virus transmission has not deterred indigenous peoples from participating in religious and traditional rituals. During the pandemic, indigenous people in this research were confronted with regulations for limiting interactions and the PPKM that are detrimental to the performance of traditional rituals, particularly those that demand greater community participation. The case of Bali and Sumba showed that the performance of traditional rituals or other festivities, which are usually drawing crowds in a particular residential area, poses a challenge to the proliferation of the COVID-19 cases.

Keywords COVID-19 pandemic · Fertility · Mortality · Population mobility · Economy · Traditional rituals

Population is an important feature of development in an area for it serves not only as the actors, but also as the objects and the beneficiaries as well. In this sense, growth and changes in the structure and composition of the population are essential aspects that must be considered from time to time. There are three essential components in the dynamics of population growth, namely births, deaths, and migration. However, the problem is that the COVID-19 pandemic has had a huge impact on social, economic, political life, and demographic dynamics throughout the world, including in Indonesia. Various studies have demonstrated that a pandemic will influence the socio-demographic conditions of a community, even in a worst-case scenario it can modify the composition of the population structure (Bender, 2018; Ridho & Yusuf, 2021).

The COVID-19 pandemic has both direct and indirect effects on various facets of life at all societal levels. Different measures set up by the government to address and manage the COVID-19 pandemic have unquestionably exerted influence over the community. Recent researches demonstrated that socio-demographic aspects are crucial to comprehending the COVID-19 pandemic, particularly as a basis for policy-making and case handling (Balbo et al., 2020a, 2020b; Kalabikhina, 2020).

According to the findings of the study, due to the duration of the pandemic, not all of the effects of COVID-19 on the demographic aspect are directly visible in a short period of time. Looking at the statistical changes, the impacts of the COVID-19 pandemic on Indonesia's demographic condition will be most likely noticeable within one or two years. However, the nearly two-year-long COVID-19 pandemic has undoubtedly had a significant impact on the trend in demography-related behavioral changes that will shape the future demographic condition of a country, including Indonesia. The wave of the COVID-19 pandemic has also a negative effect on the socio-economic condition of the population.

The most obvious demographic effect of the COVID-19 pandemic is a rise in mortality. According to data of the COVID-19 Distribution Map provided by the Committee for the Handling of COVID-19 and the National Economic Recovery, in November 2021, almost 144,000 Indonesians had died from COVID-19. Based on these statistics, the senior population (60 years and over) has the highest death rate owing to COVID-19, which is approximately 47%. Meanwhile, gender-specific statistics revealed that more males than women died from COVID-19 (52.3 and 47.7%). Other effects of COVID-19 included a drop in contraceptive use, which has the potential to increase maternal and newborn mortality (BKKBN, 2020a), and a decline in the availability of human resources in the context of population dynamics (Bender, 2018; Ridho & Yusuf, 2021). Meanwhile, Marois et al. (2020) showed that COVID-19 has also reduced life expectancy; that is, when COVID-19 prevalence rate reached at 10%, life expectancy at birth in Southeast Asia will fall by between 2 and 7 years.

When it comes to birth, several recent studies claimed that the coronavirus can directly or indirectly impair male fertility (Huang et al., 2021; Vishvkarma & Rajender, 2020). On the contrary, Dr. (HC) dr. Hasto Wardoyo, Sp.OG (K), the head of the National Population and Family Planning Agency (BKKBN), stated during a webinar session that the pandemic indirectly led to a decreasing number of contraceptives, which may have contributed to an increase in unintended pregnancies. In April 2020, it is estimated that over 47 million women in Indonesia will lose access to contraceptive services, which might lead to 7 million unplanned pregnancies (BKKBN, 2020b). This will indirectly result in an increase in birth rate. Chamie (2021) also reported that numerous developing nations, notably Indonesia, showed early signs of a baby boom, which is considered to be partly attributable to women's inability to obtain modern contraception during the COVID-19 pandemic.

In terms of population mobility and migration, the worldwide pandemic has compelled countries to regulate and close borders in order to suppress an excessive rate of infection cases. The policies have a direct impact on the community's ability to carry out normal activities, including economic and social ones. According to the Big Data of Google Mobility Reports, since the official imposition of WFH, mobility to homes and shopping centers has increased, whereas mobility to workplace has dropped. Moreover, domestic departures have decreased since the implementation of PSBB and PPKM. In addition, border crossings have been also limited. These changes in internal and international migration patterns and flows will obviously have a substantial effect on the dynamics of the Indonesian population.

The impacts of the pandemic on the social system or population, including the living system in general, will determine the response and strategy for combating the pandemic. Slightly different from the society in general, indigenous peoples have their own peculiarities and distinctiveness in living their everyday lives. Their belief in the spiritual powers of their ancestors is inherent in any activity they engage in every day. In addition to highlighting the impacts on fertility, mortality, mobility, and economy, the last part of this section will also discuss the impacts of the COVID-19 pandemic on the performance of traditional rites within the indigenous peoples at the research sites. Thus, a comprehensive account of the impacts of the COVID-19 pandemic in relation to indigenous peoples becomes possible to describe responses and strategies of adaptation during the pandemic.

4.1 Fertility

There numerous factors that may affect fertility, including cultural assumptions that "many children, many fortunes" and that children are the successors of familial and ancestral ties as well as social-economic standing. Even for inhabitants whose primary occupation is farming, increasing the family size by having more children is a viable alternative, as children are regarded a source of labor. Children can assist their parents to meet the need for workforce in completing the parents' jobs. Consequently, variations in fertility within each tribe can also be attributed to their perspectives on the importance of children within the household. From a religious perspective, children are a gift from God that should be appreciated, protected, and even unrestricted.

The Nuaulu in Central Maluku District (Maluku), the Marapu in Sumba (East Nusa Tenggara), and the Tugutil in North Maluku also cherish the importance of having so many children. For example, a girl of the Nuaulu Tribe may give birth to more than five children during her lifetime. The FGD with the women of Rohua Hamlet revealed that if they do not utilize contraceptives, the number of children born would exceed ten individuals. With knowledge of contraception, particularly a contraceptive implant, the average number of children a woman has been four to five. In the Nuaulu people, the restrictions barring intermarriage and polygamy had no effect on the rising number of marriages or potential offspring. In addition, the Matoke clan has a tendency to have a large number of children, particularly sons who are supposed to carry on the customary leadership. The husband and wife will seek to have additional children until they have a boy.

Normally, a Marapu family in Sumba has between three and four children. The pattern has remained the same during the COVID-19 pandemic. It is interesting to find that the number of children or pregnancies are determined by the women or mothers.

In this instance, the participation of women in the Marapu society (regardless of whether they have converted to a different belief) is strongly significant in shaping pregnancy and birth. The conversations with some mothers in Prailiu Village showed that the number of children began to be restricted due to the high cost of education. Those mothers want and work hard for their children to be able to attend higher levels of education. When asked for a similar information, a group of fathers gave the same answers. Pregnancy and childbearing decisions are left to the mother or woman. In the meantime, a considerable number of children can still be found in communities where their parents own a large amount of land, and their presence is intended to help their parents in the fields.

The Marapu community in both West and East Sumba limits the number of children in two ways: using traditional ingredients or contraceptives that can be obtained from the local midwife or the Community Health Service Center (*Puskesmas*). Contraception is relatively accessible to them for it can be easily received from a local midwife or a community health center. Even during the pandemic, the mothers have no reluctance to see a midwife or a health worker at the community health center, partly because they already know each other very well. Although there were worries about visiting the *Puskesmas* and other health workers at the onset of the pandemic, the situation has now reverted to normal. However, things are different when it comes to hospital visits. The people seem to avoid a visit to large hospitals due to the COVID-19 test procedure that must be completed prior to receiving medical treatment and their fears of being exposed to the coronavirus. In addition, the Marapu and the Sumba people are in general reluctant to visit the hospital because they do not know well the on-duty medical staff who are frequently coming from outside the neighborhood or even not from Sumba.

Based on discussions and interviews at the research site, Most of the Tugutil have a rather significant number of children, approximately (7–8 children). The average age of marriage is relatively young, and there are little limitations on pregnancy (natural family planning). This generation of the Tugutil, who are currently between 50 and 60 years old and have numerous offspring, were living in the forest at a young age. Meanwhile, the next generation, who are currently 20-to-40-year-old age, has begun to know health services such as contraception, resulting in a decline in the number of births (2–4 children). The forest-dwelling Tugutil people that the researchers were able to meet are between 40 and 50 years old, and their number of offspring is relatively minimal (4–5 people). Even though the Tugutil people do not receive formal health services, they claimed to be familiar with kinds of herbs that can prevent pregnancy.

Participation in the use of contraceptives was little or nonexistent among the Tugutil of North Maluku, either living in the forest or the hamlet, both before and during the COVID-19 pandemic. The majority of them do not utilize contraceptives, hence the average number of children is greater than three children per family. The forest- and village-dwelling Tugutils are drinking natural herbs from the forest to avoid pregnancy (interview with the Head of Lili Village, September 2021).

Furthermore, the response related to maternal pregnancy was similar prior to and throughout the COVID-19 pandemic. For the pregnant women living in the forest, the usual diet consists of *kasbi*, bananas, sweet potatoes, and vegetables (when anyone comes to the village), and they continue to engage in activities such as gardening and gathering despite the fact they have not yet enjoyed the services of the community health center because of its distant location unable to be routinely accessed by a health worker.

Meanwhile, the presence of integrated health service post (*Posyandu*) cadres makes the pregnancy and infant development among the village-dwelling Tugutil more closely monitored and controlled than those who reside in the forest. In addition, the health workers of *Puskesmas* often visit the hamlets (particularly Titipa and Tukur-Tukur) to give services. What has changed in Yawanli Village as a result of the COVID-19 pandemic is that in order to access public health facilities, the locals have to be vaccinated and childbirths are delivered to a community health center (Interview with the Head of the Yawanli Village, September 2021). The reason is because many Tugutil women in the Lalaici Hamlet of Yawanli Village still give birth at home with the assistance of their husbands or other family members. There has been no change in the process of giving birth for the forest-dwelling Tugutil, either before or after the pandemic; there are no health workers who accompany and assist with childbirth, and the birth process is still carried out on the outskirts of the forest, alone or with the assistance of the husband or other family members. Prior to and during the COVID-19 pandemic, the proportion of mothers and children who attended the *Posyandu* remained low. The field observations indicated that even in the village with easy accessibility, participation in *Posyandu*'s routine activities has been also minimal.

The Tengger people in Malang District (East Java) conforms to the opposite pattern regarding the significance of children. Based on the registration data, the crude birth rate (CBR) in 2021 was between 10 and 11 live births per 1,000 population. The low birth rate in Ngadas Village was because most of the people adhere to a small family norm, where the average number of children per woman is between 1 and 2, although the average age at first marriage is very young, which is between 18 to 19 years old. There is no sex preference in determining the gender of a child, nor are boys and girls treated differently in any respect.

The Tengger people intentionally restrict the number of births for economic reasons, such as fear of "*ora kopen*" and limited land. Due to their labor in the fields and the costly ceremonies for a child's birth, the women become aware of the need to join the Family Planning (KB) program to limit births. This is why the family planning program has been successfully implemented in the region. Most of them control pregnancy in modern ways by utilizing injectable contraceptives, which are obtained from health workers or centers such as midwives, nurses, and *Puskesmas*.

In an effort to continue promoting the family planning program, family planning equipment is always readily available in Ngadas Village, and the village midwife usually hosts a social event at the Posyandu once a month. The Family Planning Field Extension Officers (PLKB) and health workers promote family planning-related socialization, such as through the PKK meetings. At the sub-district level of Poncokusumo, a coaching clinic for traditional midwife (*dukun bayi*) is regularly held every month according to Javanese calendar, namely every Pon Friday (formerly on Pahing Tuesday). Outside of the Posyandu's schedule, the residents with health issues or who want to access family planning tools can contact the Village Midwife (*Bidan Desa*) through WhatsApp at any time.

Meanwhile, the Antenatal Care (pregnancy and childbirth) program for the Tengger people of Ngadas Village has been effective since 2018. This Integrated ANC program is jointly delivered by the Village Midwife and the Traditional Midwife with the support of the Poncokusumo Health Center. However, the COVID-19 pandemic has impacted services for pregnant women and toddlers, including Posyandu activities, Toddler Family Development, and prenatal classes. Due to the pandemic conditions and funding cuts, the Integrated ANC Program cannot be executed in one-hundred% performance. The program for giving contraceptives was unaffected by the pandemic; only the number of activities was reduced.

Meanwhile, the *Pethekan* tradition, which is a traditional pregnancy testing, exists to prevent unwed pregnancies among unmarried women and widows of reproductive age. This custom, which aims to control promiscuous sex among the populace, has been strongly held and obeyed. Therefore, despite the COVID-19 pandemic, the *Pethekan* tradition remains enforceable as usual.

According to the data from the Ngadas Village registration office, the number of live births for the Tengger in Ngadas Village (Malang District) tended to decrease from 27 in 2019 to 22 in 2021. This suggests that the COVID-19 pandemic has no effect on the birth rate. Information from the midwives at the Poncokusumo Health Center and in Ngadas Village revealed that the number of births in Poncokusumo Sub-District and Ngadas Village did not increase both before and after the COVID-19 pandemic.

In Sumba, particularly among the Marapu people, the COVID-19 pandemic has had no discernible effect on the rise in the birth rate. The qualitative study demonstrated that there is no increase in the number of pregnancies during the pandemic. Based on the findings of interviews and focused group discussions (FGD), no pattern of rising pregnancies was known over a period of one to two years during the COVID-19 pandemic in the research sites.

In the context of the Orang Rimba (Jambi), empirical studies conducted through interviews and focused discussions with various parties, including the local government, civil society organizations that assist the Orang Rimba, the Bukit Dua Belas National Park Office, and the Orang Rimba themselves, indicated that the pandemic situation has an impact on their conditions. Although it was hard to measure quantitatively the effect due to limited data sources, conversations with multiple parties showed that COVID-19 does not have a direct effect on the fertilities of the Orang Rimba.

Contrary to what occurs in other indigenous people, the Tengger in Ngadas Village in Malang District, the Marapu in Sumba (NTT), and the Orang Rimba in Jambi encounter a distinct phenomenon. In general, the pandemic has not had a direct effect on the birth rate; nonetheless, it is likely that the birth rate will rise in the future. This can be seen from the fact that the number of family planning acceptors did not increase nor decrease during the pandemic, or remained relatively stable.

As for the indigenous peoples of Bali, the demographic statistics showed that there are fewer new family planning acceptors per 1000 reproductive-aged couples (PUS). At the entire Bali Province as a whole, the number of new family planning acceptors declined from 71.04 per PUS in 2019 to 57.59 per PUS in 2020 (BPS, 2025). The same pattern holds true for Buleleng District. This decline indicates a possible trend toward an increase in the number of births in subsequent years.

In addition to the decline in the number of family planning acceptors, there was also a drop, although statistically insignificant, in the number of active family planning participants, particularly for pill use in Buleleng District. Regionally at the provincial level, the number of active participants increased, however the rise was not significant. Nonetheless, when measured by district, the given numbers vary, with some growing and others falling. In addition to pills, tubectomy appears to be a declining method of contraception, particularly in Buleleng District.

The drop in family planning acceptors and the continuous use of family planning devices are inseparable from the inclination not to visit health institutions such as health centers and clinics out of fear of getting COVID-19. According to many informants, visiting a health service center during a pandemic differs from regular circumstances. The high number of COVID-19 cases in their residence motivates individuals to avoid or limit visits to health care facilities.

It is true that the COVID-19 pandemic has not had a tangible impact on the birth rate among the Nuaulu; however, the tendency can be inferred from the decrease in the%age of women using family planning in Central Maluku District from 42.13% in 2018 to 39.28% in 2020 and the increase of births to four babies in the last two months. Access to contraceptives at health facilities remains regular, and participation in family planning is periodically checked. In addition to access to contraceptives, other health services such as *Posyandu* for toddlers and *Posyandu* for the elderly continue to operate during the pandemic.

A study of fertility in the Biak Numfor District in 2021 revealed an upward trend in the birth rate for the period 2010–2020, particularly during the COVID-19 pandemic that began in March 2020. The Total Fertility Rate (TFR) in Papua Province in 2020 was 2.39% higher than Indonesia's TFR, which was 2.10. Unfortunately, the birth indicator data (TFR) for Biak Numfor District is not currently available, so that the Child Women Ratio (CWR) Indicator will be used to describe the measure of reproductive history, or cumulative fertility, which evaluates the average number of children born to a woman.

According to the results of the 2020 Population Census, the CWR for Biak Numfor District in 2020 was 52.46, which is an increase from the 2010 CWR of 49.64. This implies that the fertility rate has increased during the past decade. This 2020 CWR was also higher than the Papua Province's CWR, which was only 35.16, and ranked Biak Numfor District in 13th place as the district/city in Papua Province with the highest CWR. Another interesting fact was that when the CWR of Papua Province fell throughout 2010–2020 (in 2010, it was 39.56), the CWR of Biak Numfor District climbed, and this increase occurred even during the COVID-19 pandemic in 2020.

The CWR of Biak Numfor District has declined since 2010–2019, indicating a decline in fertility rates throughout the time period. Meanwhile, the CWR increased to 52.46 in 2020, which means an increase in births. This situation demonstrates that the COVID-19 pandemic has had an effect on the demographic conditions of the Biak Numfor population, particularly on fertility indicators. The government's policy requiring people to work from home (WFH), to study from home (SFH), and restrictions on population mobility most likely contributed to this increase in fertility. In certain villages, the rate of pregnancies has risen as a result of an increase in the amount of time couples spend at home, and the phenomenon of marriages at young ages has also been linked to the lack of face-to-face educational activities for students. Considering the fact that many indigenous Papuans do not participate in the Family Planning Program (KB) due to cultural and religious concerns, this condition is clearly cause for concern. The sermons on traditional marriages preach that the OAP should reproduce as much as possible so that they do not become a minority in their own land. In addition, there are also campaigns on social media concerning the depopulation of indigenous Papuans, i.e., the decline in the proportion of Papuans to non-Papuans.

It should be noted, however, that the increase in the CWR of Biak Numfor District is not only attributable to the rising number of newborns during the COVID-19 pandemic. The occurrence of return migration that drove the Biak people to return to their village because of the pandemic has also contributed to the increase in the population of children under the age of five (0–4 years) following their parents' migration. The district with the highest CWR rate in 2020, according to the BPS data, was Orkeri, followed by Poiru, Bondifuar, East Numfor, and Warsa. In contrast, the districts of West Numfor, Oridek, East Biak, Yendidori, West Biak, Aimando Padaido, and Yawosi had CWR scores lower than the average rate of Biak Numfor District. The higher the CWR score, the higher the fertility rate, and vice versa.

4.2 Health and Mortality Rates

Morbidity and mortality are indicators that characterize a region's level of public health. Mortality is a demographic measure that serves as a means of reducing population growth. Therefore, the high and low death rates in a region represent the population health in that region. Mortality is another factor that influences the demographic makeup of a region. Consequently, the mortality rate in a region might indicate the effectiveness of the local government's efforts in maintaining the health of its population, such that life expectancy increases from year to year.

The impact of COVID-19 pandemic varies by region and can be felt directly or indirectly. The increase in positive cases and deaths of COVID-19 demonstrates the direct impact of the pandemic. In addition to raising the direct risk of death due to virus infection, the COVID-19 pandemic is believed to have increased the indirect risk of death (Roberton et al., 2020). This study also forecasts the rise in maternal and child mortality among children under the age of five as a result of probable disruptions to the health system and diminished food supply. This may happen because of the unpreparedness of the health system in facing the pandemic as well as many policies that have indirect effects on the conditions of daily living.

The results of the research on the impact of the COVID-19 pandemic on mortality and morbidity indicated that the mortality rate for COVID-19 confirmed cases tends to be low and that some indigenous populations experience loss of smell within a specific period of time (July–August 2021). Based on socio-demographic factors, vulnerability to COVID-19-related sickness and death can be described as follows:

- The population of productive age tends to be more susceptible to COVID-19 infection.
- Women are more likely to contract COVID-19.
- Older people (elderly) are at higher risk of death.
- Males account for a greater proportion of Covid-19 deaths.
- The more the movement, the greater the risk of exposure to COVID-19.
- The greater the population density, the greater the risk of COVID-19 transmission.
- The absence of health protocols among large crowds during traditional cultural/ ritual activities has the potential to facilitate the transmission of COVID-19.

According to data from the Indonesian COVID-19 Task Force, positive cases of COVID-19 in Indonesia reached 4,262,720 on December 31, 2021, with a death toll of 144,094. The fatality instances varied among provinces, with the highest number being in provinces on the island of Java, followed by other significant provinces outside of Java. When the pandemic broke out, the province of Bali was in the spotlight due to the high number of intensive tourism industries performing with no social distancing and the frequent *odalan* rituals or religious events causing crowds to gather. The national high death rate in Bali can be ascribed to the numerous crowd activities held intensively in the island. The number of deaths during the pandemic has climbed, although their reasons are still uncertain. After being exposed to COVID-19, many of those who died were already suffering from chronic illnesses or comorbidities, such as heart disease, diabetes, and other ailments. According to one of the informants, the higher mortality could be the result of a reluctance to go to the hospital, resulting in inadequate care for the type of illness suffered. Identifying the cause of death during a pandemic led to pros and cons. Some claimed that many deaths are caused by COVID-19, while others maintain that these deaths are due to the patients' co-existing diseases, such as heart attacks and abnormalities in the lungs.

Meanwhile, the data regarding the COVID-19 death tolls in Sumba are still general in nature. There are no particular information on COVID-19 deaths among the Marapu believers. Therefore, it is difficult to determine the impact of deaths associated with COVID-19 directly on this population. According to the daily monitoring data for COVID-19 cases in East Sumba, one of the research sites, as of October 8, 2021, there were 5,507 positive cases and as many as 123 deaths. East Sumba's mortality rate was approximately 2.23% (East Sumba Health Office, 2021). Sumba Island, located in East Nusa Tenggara Province, is classified as a "green zone" thanks to its low COVID-19 positive rate. The low number of COVID-19 instances does not imply that this region does not have many cases; this might be because the low testing rates are low or many individuals prefer to hide their symptoms rather than get tested for COVID-19.

The low number of COVID-19 cases in this region had an impact on the implementation of health protocols. For instance, masks were only observed in offices, stores, and highways across the city. The situation was quietly different when visiting the sub-districts where the Marapu and society in general reside. It was rare to see people wearing masks or keeping physical distance, even though the distance between houses in one village is not too far. In addition, there is one village where the houses are in groupings round-like circle that the density is fairly high. Furthermore, based on the interviews and group discussions, it can be known that the public did not receive appropriate socialization or knowledge regarding the coronavirus and its spread. Most of them knew the COVID-19 outbreak from television news and the people around.

An intriguing death-related finding concerns the typical procedure when death happens among the Sumba people in general and the Marapu in particular. It should be noted that the procession of the dead that is typically carried out does not exclusively belong to the Marapu, but also to the Sumba people in general, as this has become a sort of tradition in Sumba. The traditional death ceremony that has been adhered by the people of Sumba is a lengthy process, and it is believed that bad luck will befall the family if it is not performed. During the COVID-19 pandemic, there is a call for the dead body to be buried within three days of the date of death, whereas normally it can take between one and two years. Furthermore, in order to prevent the transmission of the coronavirus, the dead bodies of COVID-19 patients must be buried or cremated immediately, without being taken home beforehand, under strict protocols. This made people afraid and less likely to take tests or go to hospitals when they test positive for COVID-19. The fear of being intentionally diagnosed with COVID-19 (*dikovidkan*) by the hospital has become one of the hoaxes and misinformation circulating in the community. An interview with a noble or king's descendant family in Rende Village confirmed this phenomenon. Obviously, this condition can be one of the challenges in treating COVID-19 patients. On the other hand, this is a long-standing tradition or culture that has been passed down from generation to generation. In the current pandemic, a more exclusive approach is required.

In general, COVID-19 has a minor impact on the mortality rates of indigenous populations. The presence of local wisdom in each region is a contributing factor to the low number of confirmed positive cases and fatality rate. As in the Tengger people of Ngadas Village, which is very susceptible to natural catastrophes such as landslides, airflow obstruction caused by volcanic eruptions (Mount Arjuna), haze disasters (Mount Bromo), and floods (Mount Semeru). However, COVID-19 and other plagues (*pageblug*) occur very rarely. This is also the reason why the BPBD classifies Ngadas Village as a Disaster Resilient Village. The Tengger people on average live a long life and adhere to a small family norm. One of the factors contributing to their good health is their regular use of garlic, which is regarded to be a panacea for all diseases.

During the FGD, an Ngadas women described how her 8-month-old child had to be removed due to a leaking kidney she suffered during pregnancy. The infant was born healthy but was poisoned during pregnancy and, therefore, was eventually referred to a hospital in Jakarta. The mother and kid were healed, although their physical condition was poor. In this case, the midwife provided critical care until she was transferred to a hospital in Jakarta. Regarding the COVID-19 case, Ngadas Village is part of the Tengger region that is "free" of COVID-19 cases, despite the fact that the bulk of its residents do not adhere to health norms in their daily lives. According to the local people, there are no COVID-19 cases in Ngadas. Nonetheless, it seemed that the information was covered up because, as some the BPBD officials said, two residents have been diagnosed with COVID-19 and are receiving treatment at the hospital.

One of the reasons they are relatively free of COVID-19 is the high quality of their natural environment and the mobility of their people, which is not too dense because they live distant from the city and are mostly farmers. Therefore, their average movement is geared toward the exchange of agricultural products. During the PPKM period, this condition was linked with the closure of the Bromo tourism area. The residents who had businesses in the tourism industry before the pandemic shifted their attention to the agricultural sector, whose land was located within Ngadas Village, hence reducing the frequency with which they interacted with people from outside Ngadas Village. The Tengger residents of Ngadas Village are optimistic about their health. They continue to believe in the existence of the COVID-19 virus and are receptive to the vaccination policy of the government. They have their own wisdom of responding to COVID-19 that differs from the popular opinion, as seen in the Nyangoni ritual they perform as a protection against COVID-19. They are also unwilling to receive any COVID-19-related assistance, as they believed that others are in worse need. They fear that if they receive assistance, they will get the bad luck of COVID-19. Prior to the pandemic, one case of maternal mortality owing to obstetric complications occurred in 2019. In 2020–2021, there were no cases of mother, newborn, child, or other deaths due to COVID-19 or any other causes.

Likewise, the COVID-19 pandemic has affected the socio-economic and demographic situations of the Orang Rimba. Based on the empirical studies conducted through interviews and focused discussions with various parties, including the local government, civil society organizations that support the Orang Rimba, the Bukit Dua Belas National Park Office, and the Orang Rimba themselves, the pandemic situation has had an impact on the condition of the Orang Rimba, although it is difficult to measure this impact quantitatively due to the limited resources available. The impact of the pandemic on the migration of the Orang Rimba is readily apparent based on the results of interviews and observations. This section does not address the effects of the COVID-19 pandemic on demographic factors in general because, according to interviews with multiple parties, COVID-19 had no direct effect on the Orang Rimba's mortality rate. This was also explained in the subsection on the sensitivity of socio-economic and demographic conditions to the COVID-19 pandemic. This current section will investigate the impact of the pandemic on socio-demographic circumstances that are most visible in the migratory aspect, specifically the living wandering (*melangun*) pattern. The *melangun* pattern is a tradition of transitory movement for the Orang Rimba. It is also associated with socio-economic circumstances that compel the Orang Rimba to migrate.

In the Central Maluku District, COVID-19 cases increased in July 2021, and there were 63 positive cases out of 120 tests in August 2021. An interview with the Central Maluku District Health Office revealed that there were three COVID-19-related fatalities. The search found that the first individual to test positive with COVID-19 was a 40-year-old man who used to work in Ambon City. However, COVID-19 cases among the indigenous peoples, including the Nuaulu, were not properly recorded since they tended to conceal and deny having the symptoms. The Health Service noted that the government's inability to communicate with patients and their families made it very difficult to deal with the three existing COVID-19 cases. When the officers approached one of the positive COVID-19 patients in the Rohua Hamlet, the patient ran into the forest. The denial of COVID-19 came also from the patient's family, who insisted to take the positive COVID-19 patient home. There was even a case when a deceased patient who has been confirmed to have COVID-19 was buried in under traditional funeral customs with no health protocols. These cases are typically hazardous because they obscure the tracing procedure for positive COVID-19 cases. In Rounnusa Hamlet of Negeri Sepa, on the other hand, it was proven that the pandemic had not caused any deaths over the past two years, confirming that it had no effect on mortality.

Although the qualitative data on COVID-19 deaths were found, the Nuaulu's mortality rate did not increase considerably. This may indicate that the pandemic has no effect on the Nuaulu Tribe's mortality rate in Central Maluku District. Nevertheless, it is evident that this cannot be dissociated from the mistrust and denial of indigenous peoples toward the virus, for which reason not all COVID-19-related deaths were documented. In addition, this also led to the dead being buried under a funeral custom without health protocols, thereby having the potential to transmit COVID-19.

The rural and forest-dwelling Tugutil have received information about the COVID-19 pandemic. The village chiefs (*kepala desa*) serve as the information network for the Tugutil, such as those in Yawanli Village [The Orang Tugutil in Yawanli Village dwell in Lalaici Hamlet] and Lili Village [nearly all residents in this village are the Tugutil; see Chapter Two]. The chief of Yawanli Village is a village native, while the chief of the Lili Village is a Tugutil who has resided in the rural center of Lili Village. Even the chief of Lili Village had to walk all day to reach Makahar (48 km) in order to alert the local people about the COVID-19 outbreak and warn them to be wary of visitors. In addition, there are forest-dwelling Tugutil who frequently "travel down" to settlements in East Halmahera and North Halmahera (Tobelo), therefore they are aware of the pandemic known as "corona" to the Tugutil. Responses to COVID-19 for the Tugutil people, particularly those who still reside in the forest, cannot be separated from their distinct attitudes and perspectives toward death and birth. The attachment of the Tugutil people to the forest serves as the basis for their conduct, particularly in regards to health.

The tree of birth and tree of death symbolize the Tugutil's close bond with nature, especially forests and rivers. Tamalane et al. (2014) said that whenever a birth or death occurs, the Orang Tugutil will plant trees. Different types of trees are planted at birth and death. The birth tree consists of *duku* (*lansium domesticum*) and *seleguri* (*sida rhomboidea*) plants, while the death plants include a type of bamboo (*bambusa glaucescens*) and jackfruit (*artocarpus heterophyllus*). The Orang Tugutil of Makahar mark the birth of a child by placing a sign in front of their home. For the birth of a boy, a machete, a sago hammer, a water bucket, and a bow and arrow are typically shown, while a *saloi* (a rattan-made basket bag used by a woman for activities in the forest or in the garden) is displayed for the birth of a girl (Habian, Personal Communication, September 11, 2021).

Among the Orang Tugutil, particularly those who those who continue to reside in the forest, the concept of death distinct from that of the broader population. There are only two ways for them to die: by being devoured by demons (spirits) or by being poisoned; other forms of death are not recognized in their belief system (Syaiful Madjid, Personal Communication, September 14, 2021). Therefore, the Orang Tugutil will be cautious and skeptical of strangers (related to death from poisoning). Outsiders who wish to give food or drink must display both hands and taste it first. Even in the distribution of COVID-19 aid, the Orang Tugutil, particularly those living in the forest, do not want to receive assistance from strangers. The relief supplies given by the local government or personnel, for instance, must be shown to them before being accepted. One of the Orang Tugutil's strengths and strategies for avoiding the spread of COVID-19 in their society is their heightened awareness of foreigners or outsiders entering their neighborhoods.

According to the interviews and FGDs, no Tugutil died of COVID-19. In the early days of the pandemic, there have been no burials using the COVID-19 protocols. Although there is no record of COVID-19 entering the homes of the Orang Tugutil, interviews indicated that the residents of Lili Village experienced influenza and coughing between July and August. Additionally, the smell and taste senses were impaired. The symptoms were found not only in the rural center of Lili Village, but also in Makahar of km 48, Afu, and Tebin-Tebin. As there was no tracing in the form of PCR or antigen tests and the Orang Tugutil viewed them as normal, they were treated with daily consumed herbs to maintain stamina. In one week, the health of the Orang Tugutil in the village center, Makahar, Afu, and Tebin-Tebin had returned to normal.

When COVID-19 struck Indonesia, including Biak Numfor District of Papua, it attacked anyone indiscriminately: men, women, the wealthy, the poor, the aged, the young, the city dwellers, the villagers, the indigenous Papuans (OAP), and immigrants. In some instances, COVID-19 can result in death. According to data from the Biak Numfor District Health Office, the number of deaths by age is rising. The figure below shows that individuals aged 30 and older are susceptible to death when exposed to COVID-19. Many variables, including comorbidities, contributed to the increased mortality rate among individuals aged 50 and older, including those aged 50–59 years (41 instances of death) and those aged above 60 years (67 cases of death). Therefore, it is vital to intervene in the Biak Numfor people at these ages by intensifying vaccination efforts. The vaccination program is one of the community-wide efforts to enhance antibodies and attain herd immunity. Nevertheless, numerous challenges to boosting vaccination rates still exist, as there are many unfavorable perceptions about vaccines in the community, causing people to be fearful and reluctant to receive vaccinations. Furthermore, In addition, the wider public believes that Papuans' immune systems are allegedly robust due to their physical activities and natural diet.

Accordingly, the increasing number of COVID-19 cases and death rate during the pandemic were not directly proportional to the conduct of the people (both natives and immigrants) in the Biak Kota District. Based on the observations of researchers during data collection, the 3 M behaviors (wearing masks, washing hands, and keeping a distance) were not effectively applied in the community. It is true that in some crowded places, such as shops and hotels, hand washing facilities with water and soap are available. Nonetheless, in certain stands or kiosks, hardly nobody provides them. This phenomenon demonstrates that the majority of the upper middle class is aware of the dangers of COVID-19, whereas the lower middle class has not yet been adequately informed.

In Biak Numfor, COVID-19-related deaths are statistically more prevalent in urban areas; however, it is probable that many COVID-19 fatalities occur in rural areas but are not reported. This is consistent with the statement of a health worker in a particular district that COVID-19-related deaths may also occur in rural areas but it, nonetheless, remains unrecorded and unreported.

The Indigenous People of Papua believe that death is inevitable for all humans, whether through their exposure to COVID-19 or not. Consequently, there are people who believe in the existence of COVID-19 as well as those who do not. There are different religious and scientific explanations for it. For example, one informant said that "he does not believe it at all. COVID-19 is truly God's curse on humans, just as God punished the People of Noah with a flood and the people of Sodom and Gomorrah with death. COVID-19 is both a conspiracy leading up to the Third World War and God's curse on humanity. The Bible demonstrated that during the period of Noah and the Sodomites, God annihilated humanity. COVID-19 arises as a result of humankind's ever-increasing avarice on earth, which has caused environmental degradation, pollution, worldwide changes, and tremendous inequalities that have destroyed the universe. COVID-19 is God's message to mankind in the form of divine retribution. Hence, we must repent."

On the other hand, there are individuals who believe in the presence of COVID-19 yet resist vaccination for scientific grounds. One of the informants stated, "I believe in COVID-19, but I refuse to be vaccinated since I will lose my DNA before I get married. I intend to get vaccinated when I am married and have children. The vaccination must be perfectly healthy and disease-free. According to what I learned in college, there are recessive and dominant genetics. Marriage happens as a result of the collision of X variables, typically those that produce an abnormal meeting form due to a chemical charge, resulting in unsuitable shapes ranging from straight to curly and so on. Therefore, I reject vaccines not because they contradict the Bible, but because of genetic scientific concerns."

Many people do not want to be vaccinated for various reasons, including the theological belief that no vaccine will be able to cure humanity unless people repent before God. In lieu of a vaccine, the world's authorities must uphold truth and justice in order to cure humanity of the coronavirus. There is also an opinion that there is no proof that vaccinated individuals live longer than unvaccinated ones. Many individuals believe hoaxes (fake news), either originally from the Internet or word of mouth, about vaccine-related deaths. Consequently, the vaccination program in the community has been still hindered by the low participation of community, despite the involvement of religious and community leaders. The great challenge for health workers and the COVID-19 task force is to educate and socialize the population about COVID-19 using appropriate sociocultural strategies. The objective is to combat hoaxes concerning COVID-19 and deaths from vaccination with accurate information so that people become more aware of the hazards of COVID-19 and the significance of vaccines in preventing COVID-19 exposure.

4.3 Population Mobility

Indigenous populations affected impacted by COVID-19, particularly in the context of migration, may be categorized can be classified into two mayor groups. The first is indigenous individuals whose migration habits and culture are not significantly impacted by the COVID-19 pandemic and the second group consists of indigenous individuals whose movement patterns have been altered by the COVID-19 pandemic. Furthermore, under this pandemic situation, environmental resources, comprehension, and knowledge of COVID-19 have had a significant impact on migration. In addition, the government's intervention and local knowledge have also influenced the intensity of migration. This section will provide a more detailed description of the impact of COVID-19 on the plight of indigenous peoples in terms of migration. Indigenous people such the Orang Rimba, the Tengger, the Nuaulu, Bali Aga, Orang Asli Papua, the Tugutil, and the Marapu will be the primary focus of the explanation.

4.3.1 Indigenous Peoples Whose Migration is Unaffected by the COVID-19 Pandemic

- Environment and migration

The environment and beliefs influence migration out of the village and even out of the region. During the pandemic, migration has not been severely affected due to mistrust of the threats posed by COVID-19 and a desire to remain in the area. This is evident, for instance, among the Tengger, where migration is not highly intense. This circumstance exists because an increasing number of Tengger people believe that they have a moral obligation to preserve the Tengger culture in their region. The

Tengger people are bound by their culture to remain and build their region. The only motivation for migration out of or into the village is marriage.

Thus, it can be said that migration occurs through the process of marriage between the Tengger and non-Tengger individuals. If the spouse settles in Tengger, they must adhere to the practices and traditions of the Tengger in order to be recognized as a member of the tribe. On the other side, the Tenggerese's willingness to accept and welcome outsiders residing and settling in their area is evidence of their inclusive and pluralistic attitudes (Marcelo, 2021). Furthermore, by welcoming strangers and believing them to be part of the Tenggerese community, their solidarity becomes enhanced. Very low out-migration among the Tenggerese is fruit of social cohesion that exists between these groups. The primary reason for the mobility of non-permanent residents is their pursuit of further education. Population mobility is limited to small distances, remaining within the Tengger enclave, including Gubukklakah Village and Ngadisari Village.

The situation of the Tengger is not significantly different from that of the Nuaulu. The Nuaulu people have an inclination to dwell and not migrate. Ultimately, during the COVID-19 pandemic, this ailment had no direct effect on the migration of the Nuaulu population. The Nuaulu tribe community does not have a long history of migration across regions or even islands. At least, discussions concerning COVID-19 have influenced people's decisions to migrate. For the Nuaulu, COVID-19 has narrowed their space for mobility, as seen by a diminished frequency of visits to the city center of Masohi. Interviews with residents of Nua Nea Village revealed that during the peak of the pandemic, July–August 2021, it was extremely uncommon for residents to leave the village. Few individuals travel to the city center to sell their farm produce. Looking at this, the Nuaulu people seemed to have been aware of the dangers of being exposed to COVID-19 and have consequently reduced their mobility. However, they continue to engage in their regular mobility activities in the village, such as visiting a neighbor's house, searching for water, and going to the gardens around the village. The Nuaulu people have been well-informed of the threats posed by COVID-19 and have chosen to limit their mobility. Intriguingly, a bamboo-made road portal was found in Hatuhene Village, which, according to information, was used to lock the village to visitors during the peak of COVID-19. This closure is one of the strategies taken by the Nuaulu community to prevent the spread of COVID-19.

Moreover, population mobility is also related to a population's degree of reliance on other communities. In addition, the carrying capacity of the environment determines whether it has sufficient natural resources to support life. For individuals who have resources in the form of corps and who engage in forest-based activities, COVID-19 has no effect on their mobility. For example, the Tugutil people, who live both in the villages and in the forest, have not experienced any changes in the pattern or intensity of migration during the COVID-19 pandemic. The village-dwelling Tugutils maintain their regular activities, such as gardening and fishing. The Tugutils who live in the forest also carry out their usual activities, such as hunting and gathering for survival. Therefore, the connection between natural resources and the decision to not migrate is the primary determining factor. Since they have sufficient food in the forest, they do not depend on basic needs supplied from outside. The well-preserved forest areas help the Tugutils carry on their traditional customs.

The culture of semi-nomadic life continues as it was prior to the pandemic. For instance, a wife in the Gogaili valley came to the 48 kms Makahar for visiting her family. In addition, young Tugutil individuals continue to travel to villages to engage in economic activities, such as selling and purchasing forest-dwelling essentials. Moreover, the Tugutil people also keep practicing a shifting farming pattern, which has not changed throughout time. Therefore, it can be argued that COVID-19 has had little effect on the Tugutil's way of life. According to the Tugutil people who have lived in Titipa Hamlet for a long time, their forest-dwelling agricultural practices shifted at most between two areas before returning to their original location. They stayed in each farm location for approximately three months before moving to a new area for another three months and returning to the main farm and house. COVID-19 has also no substantial effect on migration for indigenous peoples who lack a migration culture, in addition to the availability of natural resources. Certainly, the availability of human resources also influences population mobility because migration also requires expertise, social networks, and a higher level of education. Seeing that the members of the Tengger, the Nuaulu, and the Tugutil prefer to reside where they were born, it can be inferred that their social networks outside the region are not well-established. On the contrary, other tribes with a nomadic culture show typically a robust social network, as evidenced by the presence of ethnic-based organizations or associations (*paguyuban*).

- Knowledge of COVID-19 and Local Wisdom

Migration decisions are primarily shaped by a combination of push and pull factors. The push factor typically comes from inadequate natural resources and the inability to sustain livelihoods. Meanwhile, the pull factor consists of the destination region being perceived to offer a more promising livelihood. The attitude of indigenous peoples to the pandemic also influenced the decision to migrate. Individuals who are not very concerned about the COVID-19 outbreak are found among the Marapu indigenous people of Sumba. Eventually, this lack of worries had no effect on their migration pattern.

Because of COVID-19, the Marapu indigenous people have also experienced mobility and migration limitations both directly and indirectly. Interestingly, the Marapu believers are not particularly worried with their normal mobility, even if it is merely between sub-districts (*kecamatan*) or districts (*kabupaten*). The people are convinced that they will be alright because their local wisdom will sustain their endurance. In addition, the belief that diseases with symptoms similar to those of COVID-19 are common during the transition season or July, which is regarded as a season of sickness, contributes to their lack of anxiety regarding this coronavirus. This perception is obviously worrisome because it suggests that COVID-19 is a common disease. On the other hand, the people attempt to maintain their immune systems by consuming herbs from leaves that have been passed down through generations. The trust toward herbal remedies that can boost the body's resistance has increased their psychological immunity. However, if not properly managed, such an understanding will make it difficult for the government to conduct tracing and testing for COVID-19, and therefore slightly hinder the implementation of health protocol policies. Thus, a sociocultural approach is needed to ensure that the government's campaign for the implementation of health regulations follows the road map that has been already set.

4.3.2 Indigenous Peoples Most Affected by COVID-19 with Regard to Migration

Each indigenous group responds to the COVID-19 pandemic differently, depending on their knowledge and understanding of the coronavirus, experience, and culture. Obviously, indigenous peoples with a long history of pandemics will be more vigilant and develop a local response system for COVID-19. The Orang Rimba are one of the indigenous peoples with a long history of pandemics. Therefore, their response was quite responsive and they did not wait for the government's orders to implement social restrictions. The same can be found in Biak Numfor, where the community put a brake on their migration activities in response to government limitations. They are also aware of the dangers of COVID-19.

- **Sensitivity and Local Wisdom in Limiting Migration**

The impact of the pandemic on the migration of indigenous people varies by environment and population. The Orang Rimba of Jambi are one of the indigenous groups whose migration patterns are affected by the pandemic. The in-migration practiced by the Orang Rimba takes the form of non-permanent migration commonly referred to as *melangun*. In fact, the philosophical meaning, length of time, distance traversed, and geographical location of the *melangun* has shifted during the pandemic. According to the interview data, the significance, distance, time period, and arena/region of the *melangun* between various groups of living environments become vastly distinct. One of the Orang Rimba we spoke with who has lived in a residential area for quite a long time said:

> The practice of *melangun* nowadays is not what it used to be. We have been living here (at home) for quite some time. Each bereaved household now does the *melangun* individually, rather than in a group. The *melangun* is carried out in a resident's garden which is not too far from the house. They just do it briefly, after that they return to their own homes. (Interview with the Orang Rimba who live in housing)

Meanwhile, some other groups living on oil palm plantations said that the timing of *melangun* cannot be determined as in the past. When a member of a group dies, the other members are unable to continue the *melangun* tradition as their elders once did. In the past, the *melangun* could be carried out across districts. If a family member dies today, especially among the Orang Rimba who reside in oil palm fields, they will leave the place and migrate (*melangun*) to a nearby area. The melangun's travel zone is limited to palm oil fields. In addition to having an effect on their customs of migration (*melangun*), COVID-19 has also had an effect on the lives of Orang

Rimba who reside in oil palm plantations. This is due to the fact that, aside from the pandemic condition, their living space to find sources of income is becoming increasingly constrained. Prior to the pandemic, it was difficult for the Orang Rimba living in oil palm plantations to meet their food and economic demands.

Due to their reduced mobility, those affected by the pandemic are unable to freely search for used goods, which has an effect on their income. In light of this circumstance, the Orang Rimba encounter hardships comparable to those of seasonal migrants, who are also more likely to miss workdays since they are unable to leave the community because of travel restrictions (Priodarshini et al., 2021). This condition cannot be avoided due to the pandemic and the Orang Rimba's inculcated understanding of the hazards of the virus, thus making the option to restrict mobility is a realistic one. Despite of all that, the Orang Rimba, particularly the forest-dwelling ones, ultimately survive by exploiting the richness of forest products.

The Orang Rimba have been wary of the outside world during this pandemic. This ailment restricted their mobility and contact with outsiders. One of the Orang Rimba in the oil palm plantation said:

> The company compelled us to switch our means of subsistence. Originally, we searched the forest for food, rattan, *jernang*, *balam*, and resin; but now where else should we go? It is finished. We are now searching for pigs and used items since that is all we can locate. There are outsiders who accommodate used items. When we scavenge discarded waste, we are occasionally suspected of theft. (Interview with an Orang Rimba worker at a Missionary Grant Palm Oil Plantation)

For the Orang Rimba who live close to the settlement, in dwellings, and on oil palm land, interactions with the broader populace are more intense. This circumstance exposes them to information sooner and makes them more susceptible, as their value system frequently conflicts with those of other residents or communities. The Orang Rimba are quite receptive in getting information, particularly from those who have experience dealing with epidemics in the past. Therefore, after getting this information, they employed a local wisdom of physical distancing called *besesandingon*.

The response of the Orang Rimba is comparable to that of the Biak Numfor, who had a migration tradition prior to the pandemic. According to the findings of the study, the Biak Numfor people were known as indigenous Papuans who used to perform migration since ancient times. Before the fifteenth century, the Biak had traversed Papua's western and eastern regions (Usmany, 2014). In the west, they sailed through Raja Ampat, Maluku, and Flores to reach the island of Java (Lapian, 2009); but in the east, traces of the Biak people have been discovered on the Sarmi coast and even in Papua New Guinea (Frank, Rumere, and lewakabessy, 2015). This is inseparable from the expertise of nature, astronomy, and sea transportation technology that they possess (Usmany, 2014). Demands of life, marital property, searches for slaves, shame, and competition (*ego korfandi*) were some of the reasons for the migration phenomena (Usmany, 2014).

However, in the current context, particularly light of the COVID-19 pandemic, we were told by a number of Biak Numfor residents that they rarely leave the village for reasons other than education. The study by Charles-Edwards et al. (2021) in Australia also predicted a 50 to 80% decrease in interstate migration between 2020 and 2021. Therefore, those who are open toward the outside world typically suffer migration pattern alterations. Normal migration patterns between cities and even between islands have shifted to migration from villages to cities. This is also true on Numfor Island. According to some residents of Kameri Village in the West Numfor District, residents from various villages in six districts of Numfor would go to the capital of the East Numfor District, which serves as the island's community hub. At the onset of the pandemic, there was an abrupt cessation of everyday local migration. According to the South Biak Presbytery Board, the mobility of people, particularly the metropolitan congregations, has been restricted on Biak Island since March 2020. Numerous roads and villages were barred, indicating that the region should not be traversed. According to one of the dealers, the Bosnik market was also blocked for up to two months following the finding of traders tested positive with COVID-19. This condition demonstrates that the people of Biak Numfor are using their knowledge and social institutions in response to COVID-19, even if they are aware that their actions may restrict their mobility and income.

In May–August 2021, which was the second phase of COVID-19 in Indonesia, the government again restricted access to the island of Numfor from the outsiders. This enforcement was accompanied by severe consequences. For the safety of residents, strict sanctions for lawbreakers in accordance with the consensus was expected to instill a sense and behavior of compliance. According to the district head of East Numfor and a church youth leader in Numfor, there were cases in which a number of Numfor locals secretly sailed to Manokwari in order to rescue their friends who were stuck in Numfor during the lockdown. However, they were caught by the island residents and authorities. In accordance with an agreement between the officers and the community, the ship was subsequently set ablaze as a form of punishment. This incident gave a lesson that consensus and decisive action are imperative to implement the government-proposed health protocols. On the other hand, the success of the campaign to preserve health protocols also depends on the support of community and religious leaders.

Numfor has started to reopen in September 2021, in which ships and aircrafts have resumed its normal operations. Prior to that, the residents of Biak Numfor were impeded in their daily migration activities as a result of restrictions placed on their mobility. In addition to blocking access roads and shutting down the markets, the security apparatus routinely conducted street raids. If someone was caught not wearing a mask, he or she would be fined. This made Biak Kota very quiet as a city of the dead in June-July 2021. It can be inferred from the description above that the migration aspect, notably among the residents of Biak Numfor, has been severely affected by the pandemic.

- The Impact of the Pandemic on Shifting Migration Patterns

One of the quite obvious migration-related consequences of the pandemic was the phenomenon of re-migration, which was one of the reasons behind the migration decision. Migration in this sense refers to the return of migrants to their areas of origin or their initial migration destination. Due to COVID-19, such migration became inevitable not only in Indonesia but also in any other parts of the world. A study by Sharma and Kandpal (2021) in India found that lockdowns had an effect on the loss of jobs, workforce, and income. This prompted people with no economic support in metropolitan areas to return to their villages. This phenomenon happens on Nusa Penida as well.

Nearly 90% of the population that had worked outside returned to their villages. The number of returning migrants in Gobleg Village was approximately 200 households, as was the amount in Pedawe Village, which was nearly the same. The return migration to villages, as occurred in the ADT and SCTPB regions, indicates a preference for employment in the agricultural sector, particularly plantations. Some of the returning migrants still possess agricultural land and plantations, enabling them to immediately utilize them as a secondary source of income during the pandemic. However, some of them were unable to use the land because it is no longer productive or because they lack access to land that they can cultivate.

Nevertheless, the return migration to the areas of origin was not the only phenomena. Even in Nusa Penida of Bali, one of the informants stated that migrants returned when tourism was booming in the 2015s. Furthermore, an informant expressed the intention to return to Kalimantan if the current pandemic did not cease, indicating that out-migration was one of the options. This condition is inseparable from the limited local resources. This tendency is also observable in Myanmar, where high rates of landlessness and low incomes have contributed to fast out-migration (Boughton et al., 2021). Therefore, land tenure is also a factor driving the population to migrate. The rate of migration can be reduced if households have multiple livelihoods as a strategy for survival when their primary source of income is no longer available (Posel & Casale, 2021). Thus, discussions on the pandemic and its effect on migration should also take the socio-economic impact into account. When the major source of income is eliminated, do people have the option to find alternative employment? In addition, social networks also determine the population's ability to withstand the circumstances caused by the pandemic.

Furthermore, the decision to migrate during a pandemic depends on the support of local resources. The research findings on the Biak Numfor indicate that delays in migration and reduced income do not always make it difficult for the OAP to meet their nutritional needs. In Anggopi village, for instance, the average OAP has their own farms. They also used to catch fish for their own consumption. During the pandemic, they can still eat from their farms and catch fish without having to purchase from the market vendors. Thus, they are able to thrive in spite of constraints and have a survival strategy that does not rely on food supply from the outside of their territory. During the COVID-19 pandemic, this condition is also seen among the Orang Rimba in the vicinity of Bukit Dua Belas National Park, where they substituted rice for tubers.

Then, once the COVID-19 pandemic wave has begun to diminish, migration activities can be performed. However, each indigenous population has a unique response; for instance, some are in direct contact with the outside world, while others are through intermediaries. The research found that in the East Numfor District, there has been a rise in the number of people leaving Numfor Island to work in the cities of Jayapura and Manokwari. According to the information provided by the District Head of East Numfor, around 2,000 individuals had migrated. They did this because economic conditions in East Numfor were not good. They moved to the city in order to work as construction laborers, dock workers, and shop owners. Some of them left with their wives and children, while others remained on Numfor Island without their families.

Meanwhile, the study on the Marapu indigenous people of Sumba revealed that in-migration happened at the research site even during the COVID-19 pandemic. There were residents in the villages of Tarung, Prailiu, and Rindi who returned home during the pandemic. According to the research findings, particularly in the last two villages, more than ten people carried out in-migration. Their return migration was mostly due to the COVID-19 pandemic, which has resulted in their jobs being terminated or no longer profitable. The majority of the returning residents were those who worked in Bali, a province severely impacted by COVID-19 for its high reliance on the tourism industry, which was the most vulnerable livelihood to the effects of the current COVID-19 pandemic. Migrants were compelled to return to their villages with little capacity to work in farms or other employment fields.

4.4 Economy of Indigenous Peoples

The COVID-19 pandemic in Indonesia has not only damaged the health of indigenous peoples, but also their economic and social circumstances. During the pandemic, indigenous populations have become one of the most vulnerable groups to the negative impacts of COVID-19. According to the United Nations Development Program (UNDP), indigenous peoples are three times more likely to plunge into poverty due to the COVID-19 pandemic (Rossa & Efendi, 2021). Out of Indonesia's 272 million inhabitants, more than seventy million belong to indigenous communities, which contribute up to Rp159.93 trillion annually to the country's economy (Rossa & Efendi, 2021). Indigenous peoples in Indonesia are dispersed in a variety of locations, each of which has distinct characteristics and different economic and cultural potential as well as social modalities.

Efforts to restrict the spread of the virus by limiting people's mobility and activities are one of the ways in which the pandemic affects the lives of individuals. Multiple local governments have enacted Large-Scale Social Restrictions (PSBB) regulations or what is now called as the Enactment of Community Activity Restrictions (PPKM) at varying levels, which are broadly enforced in all districts/cities. Consequently, this has limited the economic, educational, social, and cultural activities of the general public and indigenous peoples. Tourism is one of the activities that has been impacted by social constraints.

One of the economic activities, particularly the tourism sector, is a source of income for some indigenous peoples, such as the Tengger Tribe in East Java, the Marapu People in East Nusa Tenggara, and the indigenous Balinese. The natural and cultural wealth owned by those indigenous peoples becomes a magnet for tourists to visit the regions. Crafts such as woven fabrics, plaits, and traditional gold and silver jewelry, which had no commercial value in the Merapu people at first, have now become one of the community's economic commodities. However, the rules that restrict population mobility has rendered tourism completely inactive. The pandemic, which has been ongoing for almost two years, has had a substantial effect on the tourism industry. As a result of the COVID-19 pandemic, numerous disadvantages, such as the loss of revenue from providing lodging and vehicle rental services or selling food and handicrafts as well as the people at risk of losing their jobs, are occurring.

When the tourism industry declined, indigenous peoples relied on agricultural products from their agricultural fields and plantations. Plantation products such as potatoes, cloves, cacao, and vegetable crops help indigenous peoples live and fulfill their dietary requirements. The people of Tengger Tribe, for instance, had favored agriculture, with potatoes and cabbage as their main products, over tourism as their primary source of income even before the COVID-19 pandemic. Likewise, the Marapu people rely on animal husbandry and agriculture as a means of subsistence, with corn, cassava, and other vegetable crops being the major commodity. Because indigenous peoples who own agricultural land and plantations are able to cover their daily food requirements with agricultural and plantation items, their economic resilience is relatively stable. This has been also supported by various stakeholders, including the local government, village authorities, customary council, and most significantly, the youth movement to be involved in the agricultural sector, as is the case with indigenous peoples in Bali. The cohesion of all parties involved will eventually help the community develop a sustainable agricultural concept rooted in the local wisdom.

Indigenous peoples that rely on the tourism industry and have little agricultural land are unquestionably more economically affected. The indigenous people of Marapu, who are selling woven goods, is an example. Some weavers have begun to sell their fabrics via social media platforms or by phone to their most loyal consumers. However, sales are not the same as they were when tourism was normal prior to the pandemic. Similarly, the indigenous people of Bali suffered worse economic impacts because tourism industry has been the backbone of the regional economy.

During periods of social restrictions, people may incur economic losses. However, there has been no significant shift in the social, economic, and cultural rhythms of indigenous peoples who still live in the forest or in villages with direct access to forests, customary land, and the ocean for food supplies. The Orang Tugutil of East Halmahera District, the Orang Rimba of Jambi, and the Nuaulu tribe of Central Maluku were able to meet their food requirements through hunting, gathering, farming, and catching fish and shrimp in rivers. They are hunter-gatherers who engage in economic activities based on the trading of natural resources (Prasetijo, 2017). The economic activities of the Orang Tugutil and the Nuaulu tribe tend to be subsistence-based, which is the most basic way of life with the primary goal of survival. This lifestyle is characterized by extremely limited movement within and beyond the hamlet. Thus, the economic activities of the Nuaulu and Tugutil populations had little effect on their susceptibility to COVID-19. In fact, the pattern of life that the Nuaulu and Tugutil tribes live everyday has provided them with a high level of immunity to numerous ailments.

In contrast to the Nuaulu Tribe and the Orang Tugutil, other indigenous peoples, particularly the Orang Rimba, are subjected to a number of situations and conditions that exert significant pressure on their food security during the COVID-19 pandemic (Kristiawan et al., 2021; Suprayitno, 2021). The Orang Rimba, who depend on forest products, are having trouble meeting the demands of daily life. The forest-dwelling Orang Rimba struggles to market forest products such as jernang, rubber, rattan, and resin. In addition, the price of forest product commodities, the majority of which are export products, has fallen significantly. The sales are quite limited, and the price is low. The Orang Asli Papua (OAP) in Biak Numfor suffer a similar fate, where it is hard for them to sell their garden/fish harvests to markets in the nearby town, hence causing the people to generate lower income. However, the decline in income does not necessarily make the OAP unable to meet their basic food needs. In the village of Anggopi, for example, each OAP member on average has his or her own garden. Furthermore, they would find fish to eat. During the pandemic, they can still eat from their gardens and catch their own fish, avoiding the need to purchase food from market vendors.

Meanwhile, the Orang Rimba who reside in oil palm plantation areas are in a precarious position because, outside of the pandemic, their living space is shrinking for means of subsistence. Prior to the pandemic, it was difficult for the Orang Rimba living in oil palm plantation areas to meet their food and economic demands. In certain circumstances, clashes with the locals are inevitable. This occurs because thefts typically involve agricultural products from rural communities, Fresh Fruit Bunches (FFB) from oil palm and timber plantations, or illegal logging in protected forest regions owned by the government or corporations (Prasetijo, 2015). According to Orang Rimba, the primary reason for stealing is a lack of forest for them to live in. The Orang Rimba have gotten adequate attention from the central and regional governments as well as civil society organizations in recent years. However, the pandemic situation has complicated the transformation process. The Orang Rimba are becoming increasingly vulnerable as their living space becomes increasingly limited. Although commodity prices have decreased, especially for *jernang*, resin, and rattan, the Orang Rimba who cultivate gardens in the forest are relatively unaffected economically.

The COVID-19 pandemic necessitates that all levels of society, including indigenous peoples, are capable of adapting and implementing diverse survival techniques. Indigenous peoples receive government initiatives such as the Family Hope Program (PKH) and direct cash assistance for COVID-19, which can increase the quality of human resources, particularly in the fields of education and health, for poor family groups during the pandemic in particular. Aside from that, they also received Direct Cash Assistance (BLT) from village funds in an effort to aid their economic recovery. These initiatives from the government have been aimed to improve the economic resilience of indigenous peoples so that they can withstand the pandemic.

4.5 Observance of Traditional Rituals

The preceding subchapters have described how the pandemic condition has affected the lives of indigenous peoples, particularly in socio-demographic terms (fertility, health and mortality levels, population mobility, and economy). The following subchapter will elaborate on the impact of the pandemic on the traditional ceremonial practices at the research site.

Traditional communities or those usually referred to as indigenous people, as discussed in Chapter Two, claim to share the same historical origins and to have inhabited a certain place for generations, according to one of the definitions. In the past, indigenous peoples possessed sovereignty over land and natural resources, a sociocultural existence governed by customary laws and institutions that ensured the survival of indigenous communities. Indigenous peoples are distinguished from other societies by their preservation of cultural identity, value and knowledge systems, indigenous territories, and customary laws or institutions. Indigenous peoples have their own unique and distinctive characteristics when confronting problems or stressors, including the COVID-19 pandemic.

This subsection will begin with an examination of indigenous peoples' perspectives on the COVID-19 virus. This is essential prior knowledge, as perception will influence how an individual or group responds. Perception is an internal process that enables a person to select, organize, and interpret stimuli from his or her surroundings, and this process will impact the decisions made (Yazid, 2017). Various factors, including experience, level of education, belief system, prevalent culture, personality, level of need, and mental preparation, are believed to influence one's view of something (Sarwono, 2009; David. 2009; Erikson, 1985). Someone will estimate the presence of COVID-19 on the basis of his or her perception situations. If the stressor is perceived as threatening, an anxiety response will occur. In contrast, if the stressor is deemed non-threatening, neglect will ensue.

Based on the findings from multiple research sites, this study revealed that several indigenous informants claimed to be aware of the government's socialization of health protocols and their associated hazards. It is only that indigenous peoples, in general, do not perceive the existence of the COVID-19 virus to be a severe concern due to their lack of information and comprehension. This is what happened to the people of Asli Orang Papua (AOP), the Nualu tribe in Central Maluku, and the Marapu people in East Sumba, who see mask-wearing as a marker between "modern" or "urban" and "traditional" or "rural" cultures. COVID-19, with all of its health protocols, has separated people's knowledge into these two categories, despite that this cultural classification has no clear-cut boundaries in the day-to-day realities of life. In many cases, masks are frequently worn when accessing urban areas and their public spaces, such as shopping malls, markets, ports, airports, hospitals, health care facilities, government offices, and private firms.

The portrayal of indigenous peoples' perspectives and understanding of the COVID-19 pandemic depicts how they live in the face of the threat posed by the virus's spread. The pandemic has had a minimal effect on the observance of cultural and religious practices. Almost all traditional ritual ceremonies involved crowds and physical proximity. Based on field observations and interviews, it can be concluded that the fear of COVID-19 virus transmission has not deterred indigenous peoples from participating in religious and traditional rituals.

The indigenous people of Nuaulu tribe are an example. The Nuaulu people have not had a writing culture since ancient times, therefore their religious teachings have been passed down orally from generation to generation till the present. In living a religious life, they practice a religion with no name or have no religious texts or their equivalents. The Nuaulu tribe interprets their religious teachings through dances, music, and traditional customs. During this pandemic, the people of Nuaulu continue to engage in their traditional rituals and activities, such as the Pinamou (a coming of age ceremony for girls), the Pataheri (an initiation ritual for boys entering adulthood), and other dances such as *maku-maku*, *cakalele*, etc. Some of them believe that the symptoms caused by the COVID-19 virus only resemble runny nose and cough or seasonal respiratory ailments. Mask-wearing is likewise extremely uncommon among the Nuaulu people. They believe that masks limit breathing and that their living environment is safe from the COVID-19 threat. This feeling of safety from COVID-19 comes from the relatively low mobility of Nuaulu villagers traveling outside their hamlets. They are accustomed to gardening and hunting in the forests after which they would return to their respective homes. Even though they must leave their villages or country, it is typically for selling plantation goods and hunting trophies in Masohi City.

A similar example exists among the Tengger people, who are exceedingly obedient and stick to their traditional customs, whether in the form of major ritual ceremonies or minor festivities throughout the life cycle (Suratri, 2019). According to their beliefs, traditional ceremonies are imbued with profound meanings and values for life. By doing these rituals, they seek to achieve inwardly and outwardly protection throughout their entire lives. During the pandemic, however, they are confronted with regulations for limiting interactions and the PPKM that are detrimental to the performance of traditional rituals, particularly those that demand greater community participation. It is not easy for them to deal with this dilemmatic situation. On the one hand, they must consider government rules that restrict interactions, while on the other, they are committed to performing their traditional rituals. This appears to be the case with every indigenous population in a number of research areas, including the Tengger people in East Java, the Nuaulu people in Central Maluku, the Marapu people in Sumba, and the tribes in Papua. As an illustration, the impact of the pandemic peaked in the temporary closure of Bromo tourist area.

This condition seemingly resulted to several instances of clash between the PPKM policy regulations and indigenous beliefs. Frictions are commonplace during the pandemic. One example is the disturbing case of Tayuban (a Javanese traditional dance), which resulted in confrontation between Tengger Ngadas villagers and the local COVID-19 task force. According to local eye-witness accounts of the event, the Tayuban was held festively in front of the village head's house. Indeed, it is quite often that Tayuban is carried out at the village head's house to celebrate the Karo Momentum, which is a very sacred moment to pray for the ancestors and to foster communal harmony. In the middle of the event, the COVID-19 task force arrived to dismiss the Tayuban; the dispute then became inevitable, provoking the COVID-19 task force to disband the event unilaterally. Some local witnesses believed that even the spirits of their ancestors were not happy with this decision, thereby possessing the bodies of some locals while cursing and threatening the task force for forcibly shutting down the event. The task force backed off due to the fear and ultimately the event resumed and concluded.

Even in the midst of PPKM regulations, the Tengger people continue to hold their traditional rites while attempting to limit the number of participants without diminishing the sanctity of the rituals. Major traditional ceremonies, such as the Kasada, are still carried out by excluding participation from outside the region. In addition, the Tengger's traditional custom of assembling or *apen-apen* is not preventable even during the pandemic. Even without wearing a face-mask, they flock around the fire seeking comfort and peace. Although this traditional practice is vulnerable to COVID-19 transmission, the Tengger people culturally believes that *apen-apen* has its own health benefits. The prevailing conviction of the Tengger people, according to some local figures, is that a habit of staying up all night long as well as keeping the body in warmth will keep them well and avoid disease.

The same holds true for religious worship rituals that run as usual. For instance, in the Tengger region where Javanese Sanyata Buddhism becomes the religion of majority, communal worship is carried out every Thursday. In addition to their five daily prayers, Muslims also gather every Sunday for Friday prayers. The researcher observed the two kinds of worship and found that in the midst of pandemic routine religious services can still be carried out solemnly and without any awkwardness. Some of them were wearing a face-mask during worship while others disregarded this health protocol. Similarly, traditional rituals continued to be practiced in Bali. This is evident from the continued high demand for flowers as a religious ceremonial accompaniment.

Even more intriguing is the story of the Marapu people on the island of Sumba. The Marapu culture and beliefs are quite strong when it comes to death rituals. This has prompted the Marapu people to reject the handling of dead bodies under COVID-19 health protocols. In the Marapu culture, a deceased person may be buried for up to one or two years following death. On the contrary, the government's plea includes recommendations to bury the deceased as soon as possible, and no later than three days after the date of death, with the purpose of preserving health protocols and preventing the spread of the virus.

Meanwhile, it can be argued that the traditional and religious ceremonies of the Marapu people, excluding those associated with death, have been not heavily disturbed because the people still perform them as usual. Even in Kampung Tarung, West Sumba, November is known as Wulla Poddu, which is a sacred month for the Marapu people of Kampung Tarung. Throughout the whole month, numerous religious activities, such as weddings, circumcisions, and ceremonies for refusing reinforcements, are carried out. All these rituals are still practiced by the Marapu people of Kampung Tarung due to their loyalty and adherence to their ancestral beliefs and traditions. They believe that the failure to perform these ceremonies will bring misfortunes or punishment from their ancestors. Something similar happened also at the Prailiu traditional village and Praiyawang village in East Sumba. The Marapu indigenous people continued to perform all their religious and traditional rituals, such as marriage proposal ceremonies, weddings, stone sliding for funerals and so on.

The portrait of pandemic situations full of limitations is also seen among the indigenous people of Bali. The performance of traditional rituals or other festivities, which are usually drawing crowds in a particular residential area, poses a challenge to the proliferation of the COVID-19 cases. According to some news, traditional rituals have become one of the clusters responsible for the rapid spread of the virus. Efforts to control the spread of the virus in Bali are carried out by issuing working papers that put restrictions on activities including customary ones. For example, the Governor of Bali published a Circular Letter No. 07 of 2021 pertaining to the extension of village/ward-based PPKM, which was then followed by a circular letter from the Parisada Hindu Dharma (PHDI) and the Traditional Village Council (MDA) No. 076/PHDI-Bali/VIII/2021 regulating the types of ceremonies permissible for the Balinese Hindu community to perform. When the PPKM level 4 was implemented, the number of participants in traditional rituals, such as funerals and weddings, was restricted to a maximum of ten individuals. Activities that would be normally held communally were strongly recommended to take place in each house's family temple. In conjunction with the renewal of the PPKM Level 4 in Java and Bali, the Parisadha Hindu Dharma Indonesia (PHDI) of Bali and the Bali Provincial Traditional Village Council (MDA) issued circular letters regarding restrictions on traditional ceremonies. The Circular Letter No. 076/PHDI-Bali/VIII/2021 and the Circular Letter No. 008/SE/MDA-Prov Bali/VIII/2021 regulate all forms of ceremonies in the Panca Yadnya (five types of sacred offerings devoted to Dewa Yadnya, Pitra Yadnya, Rsi Yadnya, Manusia, and Butha Yadnya) to be carried out very strictly and limitedly (Bali Channel, 2021).

Death processions also has the potential to bring crowds. A modest procession, however, can prevent a great deal of participation from the crowds and intense physical and social contacts. In addition to it, there seems to be a difference between the Bali Aga community and the Balinese communities in general in terms of religious rituals held routinely according to the Balinese calendar. The Bali Aga community has a lower intensity of religious rituals because all their religious events are consolidated into one massive major event once every two years. The observance of this traditional ceremony every two years has a profound significance for both the preservation of nature and social harmony.

The situation is not much different in Papua. The Indigenous Papuans continue to believe that being reported as having been tested positive for COVID-19 is a disgrace to their extended family and therefore should be avoided. There seems to be ambivalent or dual perceptions and attitudes with regard to the coronavirus. The Orang Asli Papua (OAP) who have never experienced COVID-19 and reside in rural areas are generally unconvinced of its existence. Nevertheless, when they learn that someone in their village have been exposed to COVID-19, they will avoid the area to prevent its spread. On the one hand, they deny the presence of COVID-19, yet when the virus arrives, they choose to keep away rather than taking a greater risk.

COVID-19, by implication, has become a sensitive term in the knowledge of Orang Asli Papua. When asked whether COVID-19 is present in the town, an informant responded by having to claim "There is no COVID-19" despite the positive symptoms declared by the hospital; admitting the presence of the virus, he said, would only raise pros and cons. In fact, when uttering the term "COVID-19," one must pronounce it very slowly or use the word "that disease (*penyakit itu*)." There was a case when a woman who tested positive for COVID-19 at the Puskesmas was asked to isolate herself. The patient received the antigen test results and urged the Puskesmas to keep her disease under wraps. The Puskesmas granted her request and instructed her to carry out self-isolation at home and to wear a face-mask at all times. We were startled to learn from the Biak Health Service's official report that this patient was walking around her village as usual.

The religious aspect is another reason behind the Orang Asli Papua's denial of the existence of COVID-19. Many informants, especially those living in rural areas and on islands, relayed this information. A tribal chief of Yawosi (HR) said that he "does not believe at all" in COVID-19. In his opinion, COVID-19 is a sort of God's curse on humankind, similar to what God did to the people of Prophet Noah (Noah) with a worldwide flood or to the people of Sodom and Gomorrah with a mass extinction. The current pandemic arose as a result of the avarice of modern humans, who have caused catastrophic damages to the universe in the form of ecological devastation, climate change, and a yawning gap between the rich and the poor. Furthermore, COVID-19 is a global political conspiracy before the coming of a greater war and this pandemic will eventually lead to an even greater catastrophe, namely World War III. Thus, the tribal chief (*mananwir*) envisaged the COVID-19 pandemic as a manifestation of God's wrath against sinful humanity and a divine command for all people to recognize their sins and to repent. COVID-19 can be averted by multiplying prayers, worships, and good behaviors toward the fellow human beings and the universe as well as spreading peace and compassion among God's other creatures. Vaccines will not cure humanity of the pandemic, he claims, but "repentance" and the world's leaders upholding truth and justice will.

References

Balbo, N., Billari, F. & Melegaro, A. (2020a). The strength of family ties and COVID-19. Contexts, American Sociological Association.

Balbo, N., Kashnitsky, I., Melegaro, A., Meslé, F., Mills, M.C., de Valk, H., & de Vilhena, D.V. (2020b, Mei). Demography and the coronavirus pandemic. https://www.population-europe.eu/files/documents/pb25_COVID-19.pdf

Bender, L. C. (2018). Age structure and population dynamics. In *Encyclopedia of ecology* (2nd ed., Issue October 2017). Elsevier Inc. https://doi.org/10.1016/B978-0-12-409548-9.10925-X

BKKBN. (2020a). Strategi mencapai target RPJMN 2020–2024 bidang kependudukan di Era COVID-19 dipresentasikan oleh Kepala BKKBN pada Webinar Indonesian Demographic Outlook 2021. [22 Desember 2020].

BKKBN. (2020b). Situasi terkini penggunaan kontrasepsi masa pandemi COVID-19. Webinar Indonesian Demographic Outlook 2021. [22 Desember 2020]. https://dktindonesia.org/wp-content/uploads/2020/09/Materi-Deputi-KBKR-DKT-final.pdf

Boughton, D., Goeb, J., Lambrecht, I., Headey, D., Takeshima, H., Mahrt, K., Masias, I., Goudet, S., Ragasa, C., Maredia, M. K., Minten, B., & Diao, X. (2021). Impacts of COVID-19 on agricultural production and food systems in late transforming Southeast Asia: The case of Myanmar. *Agricultural Systems, 188*(September 2020), 103026. https://doi.org/10.1016/j.agsy.2020.103026

BPS. (2025). Banyaknya Pasangan Usia Subur, Akseptor Baru, dan Klinik Keluarga Berencana Menurut Kabupaten/Kota di Provinsi Bali. https://bali.bps.go.id/id/statistics-table/1/MTE2IzE=/banyaknya-pasangan-usia-subur--akseptor-baru--dan-klinik-keluarga-berencana-menurut-kabupaten-kota-di-provinsi-bali--2019-2024.html

Chamie, J. (2021). COVID-19 Pandemic: Demographic highlights. *IUSSP Online News Magazine.* https://www.niussp.org/health-and-mortality/COVID-19-pandemic-demographic-highlights/

Charles-Edwards, E., Wilson, T., Bernard, A., & Wohland, P. (2021). How will COVID-19 impact Australia's future population? A scenario approach. *Applied Geography, 134,* Article 102506. https://doi.org/10.1016/j.apgeog.2021.102506

Frank, S. A. K., Rumere, J., & Lewakabessy, B. (2015). *Persebaran Orang Biak di Kepulauan Komamba SARMI-Papua.* Bala Pelestarian Nilai Budaya Jayapura-Papua.

Huang, C., Ji, X., Zhou, W., Huang, Z., Peng, X., Fan, L., Ge, L., & Zhu, W. (2021). Coronavirus: A possible cause of reduced male fertility. *Andrology, 9*(1), 80–87. https://doi.org/10.1111/andr.12907

Kalabikhina, I. E. (2020). Demographic and social issues of the pandemic. *Population and Economics, 4,* 103. https://doi.org/10.3897/popecon.4.e53891

Kristiawan, J., Prasetijo, A., & Sutiningsih, D. (2021). Ketahanan pangan KKeluarga Orang Rimba Selatan Taman Nasional Bukit Dua Belas Jambi: Studi mikroetnografi keluarga Njalo dalam menghadapi pandemik. *Jantro, 23*(1). https://doi.org/10.25077/jantro.v23.n1.p83-92.2021

Lapian, A. B. (2009). *Orang laut, bajak laut, raja laut: Sejarah kawasan Laut Sulawesi Abab XIX.* Komunitas Bambu.

Marcelo, G. (2021). Transnationalizing recognition: A new grammar for an old problem. In G. Schweiger (Ed.), *Migration, recognition and critical Theory. Studies in Global Justice* (Vol. 21). Springer, Springer Nature. https://doi.org/10.1007/978-3-030-72732-1_4

Marois, G., Muttarak, R., & Scherbov, S.(2020). Assessing the potential impact of COVID-19 on life expectancy. *Journal Plos One.* https://doi.org/10.1371/journal.pone.0238678

Posel, D., & Casale, D. (2021). Moving during times of crisis: Migration, living arrangements and COVID-19 in South Africa. *Scientific African, 13,* Article e00926. https://doi.org/10.1016/j.sciaf.2021.e00926

Prasetijo, A. (2015). *Orang Rimba, true custodian of the forest: Alternative strategies and actions in social movement against hegemony.* Jakarta: ICSD (Indonesia Center for Sustainable Development) & KKI WARSI (Komunitas Konservasi Indonesia WARSI).

Prasetijo, A. (2017). Livelihood transformations of the Orang Rimba as tacit resistance in the context of deforestation. *Endogami: Jurnal Ilmiah Kajian Antropologi, 1*(1), 1. https://doi.org/10.14710/endogami.1.1.1-13

Priodarshini, R., Biswas, B., Sánchez Higuera, A. M., & Mallick, B. (2021). Livelihood challenges of 'double strike' disasters: Evidence from rural communities of southwest coastal Bangladesh during the Covid-19 pandemic and cyclone Amphan. *Current Research in Environmental Sustainability, 3,* Article 100100. https://doi.org/10.1016/j.crsust.2021.100100

Ridho, S. L. Z., & Yusuf, S. A. (2021). Dinamika komposisi penduduk: Dampak potensial pandemi COVID-19 terhadap demografi di Indonesia. *Populasi, 28*(2), 32–53. https://doi.org/10.22146/jp.63351

Rossa, V., & Efendi, A. D. (2021). UNDP: Masyarakat adat berisiko 3 kali lebih besar menjadi miskin akibat pandemi COVID-19. Suara.com. https://www.suara.com/lifestyle/2021/12/18/123117/undp-masyarakat-adat-berisiko-3-kali-lebih-besar-menjadi-miskin-akibat-pandemi-covid-19

Sharma, R., & Kandpal, V. (2021). COVID 19 pandemic and international migration: An initial view. *Sustainable Operations and Computers, 2*(June), 122–126. https://doi.org/10.1016/j.susoc.2021.06.002

Suprayitno, T. (2021). Nasib Orang Rimba: Selamat Dari COVID-19 Tapi Kelaparan di Dalam Hutan. https://projectmultatuli.org/nasib-orang-rimba-selamat-dari-COVID-19-tapi-kelaparan-di-dalam-hutan/

Tamalane, M. N., Al Muhdar, M. H. I., Suarsini, E., & Rochman, F. (2014). The practice of local wisdom of Tobelo Dalam (Tugutil) tribal community in forest conservation in Halmahera Indonesia. *International Journal of Plant Research, 4*(4A), 1–7. https://doi.org/10.5923/s.plant.201401.0

Vishvkarma, R., & Rajender, S. (2020). Could SARS-CoV-2 affect male fertility? *Andrologia, 52*(9), Article e13712. https://doi.org/10.1111/and.13712

Chapter 5
The Strategies of Indigenous Community in Dealing with the Pandemic

Anggi Afriansyah, Inayah Hidayati, and Muhammad Saifullah Rohman

Abstract This chapter consists of three sections that describe the strategies of indigenous people in dealing with the COVID-19 pandemic. Indigenous peoples adapt in numerous sectors, including the social, economic, and cultural fields. Indigenous people make some adjustments and methods to deal with uncertainty posed by the pandemic. Additionally, a synergy between individuals, communities, and government agencies is a crucial component in response to the pandemic. This chapter attempts to illuminate the strategies employed by indigenous peoples in answering, overcoming, and adapting to the numerous changes. Afriansyah et al. illustrate that a number of indigenous peoples have their own local knowledge that defines their identity as indigenous peoples in response to the COVID-19 pandemic in Indonesia. They do not see the emergence of the COVID-19 pandemic in Indonesia and the rest of the world solely from a health standpoint, but also holistically through the lens of their local wisdom and culture in the face of the pandemic. Certain indigenous peoples, for instance, believe that COVID-19 is also a God-created thing; thus, humans must be able to coexist with it. This pandemic condition caused by exposure to COVID-19 requires prudent action. Most Indigenous peoples continue to rely on traditional medicinal knowledge as an integral part of their daily lives. However, indigenous peoples perceive and address the COVID-19 pandemic not only from a medical standpoint but also from a spiritual and cultural perspective. Various indigenous peoples at the research site also carry out a number of traditional rituals or ceremonies to shield their territory and people from the transmission of COVID-19. Moreover, there are strategies in the socio-economic-cultural domain during the pandemic. In the education part, the teachers are regularly visiting their students

A. Afriansyah (✉)
Research Center for Population, National Research and Innovation Agency (BRIN), Jakarta, Indonesia
e-mail: anggi.afriansyah@brin.go.id

I. Hidayati
Directorate for Human Development, Demography, and Culture Policy, National Research and Innovation Agency (BRIN), Jakarta, Indonesia

M. S. Rohman
Research Center for Society and Culture, National Research and Innovation Agency (BRIN), Jakarta, Indonesia

C. Pamungkas et al. (eds.), *The Impact of the Pandemic on Indigenous People in Indonesia*, Quality of Life in Asia 20, https://doi.org/10.1007/978-981-96-4222-9_5

to teach. The coping strategies adopted to address economic difficulties during the pandemic entail optimizing agricultural and plantation activities. For example, the agricultural sector is most likely to absorb migrant workers returning to Bali. Some of them are working on land owned by their families, while others are cultivating someone else's land or becoming hired labor.

Keywords Indigenous people · COVID-19 pandemic · Response · Adaptation · Local knowledge

The COVID-19 pandemic has posed challenges for the rights of citizens to health and life. More than 100 countries have announced emergency situations and measures in response to the pandemic (The Committee for the Coordination of Statistical Activities, 2020). The pandemic situation affected almost all people around the world and indigenous peoples are no exception. According to multiple reports, indigenous peoples lack access to essential services such as health, sanitation, clean water, soap, and disinfectants, as well as preventative measures against communicable and non-communicable diseases. Furthermore, indigenous populations are susceptible to stigma and discrimination (United Nations, 2020).

The advent of a health crisis due to the COVID-19 pandemic reaffirms the significance of indigenous food systems designed for indigenous peoples by their predecessors to address existing difficulties such as conquests, wars, diseases, pandemics, and climate changes (Lugo-Morin, 2021). With limited access to facilities and services, indigenous peoples must devise a strategy to fight against a pandemic. Indigenous peoples are employing every available resource to counteract this pandemic. For instance, local and cultural knowledge in each indigenous group is one of the keys to dealing with the pandemic. In some indigenous populations, the usage of herbal medicines and local potions is considered effective to prevent a pandemic (Iwuoha & Aniche, 2020). Indigenous peoples adapt in numerous sectors, including the social, economic, and cultural fields. They make some adjustments and methods to deal with uncertainty posed the pandemic. Additionally, a synergy between individuals, communities, and government agencies is a crucial component in response to the pandemic. This chapter attempts to illuminate the strategies employed by indigenous peoples in answering, overcoming, and adapting to, the numerous change.

5.1 Indigenous Peoples' Local Wisdom and Culture in the Face of the COVID-19 Pandemic

Indigenous peoples are individuals who rely on a variety of local wisdom and culture in living their daily lives. Usually, local wisdom is passed down and retained for generations by the ancestors. This local genius is then used in a manner that reflects the harmony with fellow humans and the cosmos as well. Because it is an intrinsic part of indigenous peoples' daily life, this local wisdom is preserved. We can also say that indigenous people in a given region have viewpoints, insights, and ideas concerning their environment, all of which can be defined as local wisdom (Kristiyanto, 2017). Local wisdom consists of local beliefs that are wise, insightful, and full of values firmly entrenched and followed by the community members (Rumilah et al., 2020). Local knowledge that flourishes and grows at the heart of its support community throughout the archipelago is a cultural wealth that must be cultivated (Nasruddin, 2010). This local wisdom constitutes the basis upon which the cultural identity of its support community is formed.es brought about by the COVID-19 pandemic. This chapter will discuss the following topics: (i) indigenous peoples' local wisdom and culture in addressing the COVID-19 pandemic; (ii) adaptation strategies in the socio-economic-cultural field during the pandemic; and (iii) the synergy between indigenous peoples and local governments in dealing with the pandemic.

Similarly, in response to the COVID-19 outbreak in Indonesia, a number of indigenous peoples have their own local knowledge that defines their identity as indigenous peoples. This local knowledge has a far broader scope than traditional knowledge alone (Kristiyanto, 2017). They do not see the emergence of the COVID-19 pandemic in Indonesia and the rest of the world solely from a health standpoint, but also holistically through the lens of their local wisdom and culture in the face of the pandemic. Certain indigenous peoples, for instance, believe that COVID-19 is also a God-created thing, thus humans must be able to coexist with it. This pandemic condition caused by exposure to COVID-19 requires prudent action. The Javanese people, for example, have the ability to understand specific signs or natural characters (*tetenger*), the usage of herbal medicine, and the performance of heirlooms cleansing rituals, all of which has become a cultural mechanism handed down for generations (Rumilah et al., 2020). The following are examples of indigenous peoples' local wisdom identified from our research sites:

(a) Knowledge of traditional medicines and plants for health

There is no indication that COVID-19 will be gone by 2022, and there are even multiple new virus strains. Strict health protocols have been implemented by the government and the community to stop the spread of the virus. Some health professionals are also searching for medications and vaccinations to bring the virus down. In addition to the medical efforts, people enhance their stamina by consuming alternative (traditional) remedies derived from traditional plants. For example, the tradition of ingesting herbal medication (*jamu*) has been an inherent part of Javanese local wisdom (Rumilah et al., 2020). In fact, Indonesia has been known as a tropical country with a great variety of plants. Based on their knowledge and experience, indigenous peoples are usually using some of these plants as remedies to cure certain illnesses. On the other hand, herbs produced from plants growing in Indonesia can be utilized as herbal ingredients to boost the immune system. Since ancient times, Indonesian forefathers have utilized the country's biodiversity as traditional medicines. Indonesia is recognized for its wealth of knowledge on traditional medicine and plants. It should be mentioned that indigenous Indonesians have a greater understanding of drugs and medicines than indigenous tribes in Thailand (Daulay, 2012).

Most of indigenous peoples continue to rely on traditional medicinal knowledge as an integral part of their daily lives. The understanding of medicine and treatment is one of the most essential feature of traditional knowledge (Daulay, 2012). In the province of Jambi, for instance, the members of Orang Rimba who reside in oil palm plantations still believe and count on their hereditary traditional methods for their protection against COVID-19. They believe that particular kinds of sugar cane tree will be able to shield their environment from COVID-19 and other diseases. According to Setyowati's research (2003), in the area of Bukit Dua Belas there are 195 species of plants beneficial for life, all of which can be used for food ingredients (69 types), for medicinal materials (39 types), for household appliances (11 types), for building materials (42 types), for ritual events (9 types), for rubber-producing (5 types) or for tuba and ropes-making (others). All of this is certainly in favor of the indigenous people's knowledge of traditional medicinal plants.

A similar situation exists in Biak-Numfor of Papua, where local indigenous people continue to use traditional medicines to boost their immune systems against the COVID-19 virus. When the body's immunity increases, COVID-19 will not enter the body. Herbal medicine to treat disease and enhance general health is usually produced from the abundant biodiversity (Daulay, 2012). Since COVID-19 has begun to spread in Papua, people have attempted to relearn aspects of traditional medicine that, before the pandemic, had been largely forgotten along with the development of the modern health sector. Therefore, some members of the Orang Asli Papua have returned to using the leaves or roots of trees for treatment of diseases. In the past, people bathed in seawater to eliminate smallpox, and this practice is being revived during the current pandemic. In certain indigenous peoples, traditional knowledge on medicinal plants and immune-boosting practices have been passed down from generation to generation.

The indigenous people of the Nuaulu tribe in Maluku are also well-versed in traditional medication and treatment. They still depend on forest products to supply their basic needs, including medicine. They have valuable local knowledge of how to utilize plants for medical purposes (Kotala & Firdhausi, 2019). They are also familiar with numerous leaves, plants, and even fruits that can be used to treat various ailments. They use different kinds of leaves to cure certain illnesses, such as starfruit leaves for high blood pressure, jatropha leaves for heat, biana leaves for boils, itchy leaves for weariness, cogongrass (the roots) for malaria, and unfurled leaves for fever. Kotala and Firdhausi's study (2019) recorded that as many as 31 species of medicinal plants belonging to 22 families have been used by the Nuaulu tribe in Rohuwa Hamlet of Sepa Village.

(b) Customary rites/traditional ceremonies for protection from COVID-19

Talking about indigenous peoples cannot take place without considering ceremonies or rituals, especially those relate to the human life cycle, such as birth, marriage, and death. In view of the COVID-19 pandemic, it is safe to say that indigenous peoples are somewhat distinct from the broader public. In an effort to reduce disaster risks, rituals are performed, particularly when dealing with a pandemic (*pagebluk*) (Rumilah et al., 2020). Indigenous peoples perceive and address the COVID-19 pandemic not only from a medical standpoint, but also from a spiritual and cultural perspective. Various indigenous peoples at the research site also carry out a number of traditional rituals or ceremonies to shield their territory and people from the transmission of COVID-19.

Nyangoni is an example of a traditional ritual carried out by the indigenous people of Tengger in Malang District, East Java. The Tengger people of Ngadas Village, Poncokusumo Sub-District of Malang District are building a fortress of spiritual strength to ward off the spread of COVID-19. Being a mountainous Javanese community that has existed since the Singosari era and developed during the Majapahit times, the Tengger People keep a firm hold of the teachings of their forefathers and ancestors, which foreground respect for one's fellow humans, nature, teachers, traditional leaders, government, and *Hong Pikulun*, the Lord of the universe. The Tengger People considers harmony between humanity, nature/environment, and supernatural powers—*Hong Pikulun*, the guardian gods of Bromo, and ancestor spirits—to be the ideal way of life (Radhia, 2021).

The Tengger people also revere the "earth" as the ground on which we stand and life sustains. The earth and everything on it are gifts from God Almighty, but it can a blessing or a curse on human life. Consequently, the *slametan* ritual is frequently performed to pay homage to and maintain human relationships with the earth, the environment, and the universe. When performing a Tenggerese ritual, for instance, the shaman never exclude the word "motherland (*pertiwi*)" in his mantra because it is so important for their lives (Radhia, 2021). The Tengger people of Ngadas Village believe that living in harmony with other God's creatures is an ancestral teaching that they always hold fast.

As a cultural and religious response to COVID-19, the Tengger people of Ngadas hold a ritual ceremony of *nyangoni*. According the village chief, the village chief's mother, and local religious leaders, the *nyangoni* ceremony is staged by gathering all people in the village chief's yard. The ritual begins with a prayer led by each religious leader of different religions (Buddhism, Hindu, and Islam) and then continues according to customary practices under the direction of a shaman. The philosophy of *nyangoni* says that COVID-19 is analogously nothing more than a God's creature, and in order to prevent it from entering Ngadas village, it must be given supplies (*disangoni*) by which it can continue its own journey and hopefully will be only passing through Ngadas. *Nyangoni* represents a form of gratitude from the people by which diseases and disasters are expected to leave after having been pocketed with thankful goods and offerings (Muchammad et al., 2021).

In addition to the nyangoni ritual carried out communally by the Tengger people of Ngadas village, the shaman (together with his assistants: *pak sepuh* and *pak legen*) performed a private rite to protect Ngadas Village from the COVID-19 virus. The shaman, with help from *pak legen*, held a traditional ritual of fencing the village. The shaman asked *pak legen* to collect holy water from the *widodaren* and *wendit* springs, which were mixed into one and placed in a jug. Then, at twelve o'clock in the evening, the shaman and *pak legen* walked around the village while sprinkling the water at every T-junction road of Ngadas Village. The water itself represents a source of life and is viewed as a medium that safeguards the lives of villagers from all threats and illnesses that can harm human existence. For the Tengger people of

Ngadas Village, COVID-19 is not something that should be rejected because it is also a "being" created by God; instead, humans must live in harmony with it by maintaining a good relation with it.

Other indigenous peoples held a ritual of *tolak bala* (ward off misfortune) to avoid the spread of COVID-19. The ritual of *tolak bala* seemingly finds it relevance during a pandemic crisis so that it is pursued with the expectation that the disease would cease soon and life will return to normal (Rumilah et al., 2020). The indigenous people of Marapu in East Nusa Tenggara are among those who celebrate the ritual of *tolak bala.* As a distinct community, specifically as the followers of Marapu belief, they conceive that the outbreak of the COVID-19 pandemic occurs due to many Marapu believers abandoning their faith. Apart from the matter of belief, the increased rate of immorality and misconducts, such as promiscuity among teens, in contemporary societies caused the Earth to maintain its balance by releasing a new virus that remains uncertain when it will come to an end.

Such a realization subsequently prompted the efforts to end as soon as possible the COVID-19 pandemic in Indonesia through practices of *tolak bala* or prayers. However, the indigenous people of Marapu have not yet performed the ritual of *tolak bala.* The event was indeed scheduled to take place in 2020 (particularly in Praiyawang). However, it was cancelled because some corpses had not yet been buried, which became a hindrance to a flawless performance of traditional ceremonies. Meanwhile, a traditional ceremony called *Wula Pollu* was to be held in October–November in Tarung Village. This traditional ritual was going to involve all components of society and was open for public to attend. The purpose of traditional rites such as the *Wula Pollu* is to beseech God Almighty for blessings and safety (for the followers of the Marapu belief).

The indigenous people of Bali, particularly in Munduk Village, also performed a ritual to ward off misfortunes. *Bendesa* (the traditional village chief) plays a key role in coping with COVID-19 in Munduk Village, which is part of Catur Desa Adat Dalam Tamblingan. The *bendesa* serves not only as a member of a Mutual Cooperation Task Force (Satgas Gotong Royong) that strives to induce compliance with health protocols, but also conducts numerous rituals of tolak bala. For them, the Seen (*Sekala*) as materialized in the establishment of the Task Force must be balanced with the Unseen (*Niskala*) through the practices of *pengaci-acian* in dealing with COVID-19. During the pandemic, the *bendesa* of Munduk Village was recorded to have carried out the ritual of *pengaci-acian* ten times in order to fend off any bad luck brought by the virus. Furthermore, *bendesa*, through *pecalang* (Bali's traditional guards), strictly supervises religious ceremonies and traditional processions that have the potential to attract huge audiences, limiting them to a maximum of fifteen participants. Dane Pengrajeg, the top leader at Catur Desa Adat Dalam Tamblingan, was the one who made the decision to limit religious events and traditional processions, stating that God undoubtedly will understand the choice to limit the performances of traditional ceremonies for pandemic concerns. As the primary source of legislation, Dane Pengrajeg's ruling on restricting ritual activities offers assurance for all individuals within Catur Desa Adat Dalam Tamblingan to stay in compliance.

Another type of traditional ritual or ceremony is *Usi Rosa*, which is practiced by the Nuaulu indigenous people of Maluku. The Nuaulu people of Rohua staged the *Usi Rosa* ceremony in October 2020 to prevent the spread of COVID-19 in their region. The *Usi Rosa* is a traditional procession aimed to atone for sins. It was joined by all grown-up residents of Rohua who still adhere to the religious beliefs of the Nuaulu tribe. More than 100 Rohua locals participated in this large-scale mass gathering. In addition to *Usi Rosa*, some other rituals, including *Maku Maku* and *Cakalele* dance, must be performed. During that time, the *Usi Rosa* ceremony was also staged in the hope that the people of Rohua will be spared from a variety of plague, including COVID-19. The Nuaulu indigenous people of Rohua believe that there is a close relationship between the multitude of sins and disease outbreaks. Therefore, the pursuance of the *Usi Rosa* takes on greater significance during the pandemic. According to a local community leader, "The Almighty knows that those who make the greatest mistakes will suffer the most diseases" (Hamlet Apparatus, personal communication, 9 September 2021).

(c) Customs and traditions of indigenous peoples for self-protection and immunity and health enhancement

Customs and traditions are noble values that indigenous peoples strive to maintain because of their significance in defining their indigenous identities. These are also what set them apart from other communities. Some customs and traditions are still observed by indigenous communities, showing actually that during the pandemic they serve as a self-defense mechanism against the spread and transmission of the coronavirus. The historical experiences of indigenous people in coping with life phenomenon in the past might have exerted a great influence to the establishment of customs and traditions as well as their continued observance in daily lives.

We can take a look at how the Orang Rimba keep their local wisdom alive over generations, such as the *melangun* tradition that continues to this day. The *melangun* is a tradition that determines the identity formation of the Orang Rimba as an ethnic group distinct from other communities in Jambi (Kristiawan et al., 2021). In the past, *melangun* was described as a period of migration caused by the death of a member of the group (Prasetijo, 2017). The Orang Rimba instantly fled the settlement after someone in their group was died (Prasetijo, 2017). The duration of *melangun* in the past could be years (it could even go up to seven years) (Steinebach, 2012). During the Case Session No. 35/PUU-X/2012 that involves a Judicial Review of Law No. 41/1999 on Forestry Against the 1945 Constitution of the Republic of Indonesia, Tumenggung Tarib (2012) also highlighted the philosophy, length of time, distance traveled, and location of the *melangun*. According to him, in ancient times the *melangun* could last for ten to twelve years; however, because the area of *melangun* has turned into a corporate zone and Bukit XII National Park, the time span for *melangun* is now between four months and one year.

The distance traveled for *melangun* is becoming shorter; in addition, the *melangun* is now mandatory only to the members of the deceased's family rather than to all members of the group. The increasingly narrow areas of mobility for the Orang Rimba contributed to this new pattern of *melangun*. During the pandemic, major shifts are taking place in the tradition of *melangun* in terms of its philosophical significance, length of time, distance traveled, and location, which according to the interviews have become extremely diverse between the groups of different living spaces. One of the Orang Rimba who has been living in housing for an extended period of time said:

> The practice of *melangun* nowadays is not what it used to be. We have been living here (at home) for quite some time. Each bereaved household now does the *melangun* individually, rather than in a group. The *melangun* is carried out in a resident's garden which is not too far from the house. They just do it briefly, after that they return to their own homes. (Interview with the Orang Rimba who live in housing)

Whereas, other groups inhabiting oil palm lands asserted that unlike in the past, it has been hard now to draw a definite time for *melangun*. When a member of group dies, the rest is no longer able to exercise the *melangun* tradition in the same way as their parents once did. When a family member dies, they will leave the area and migrate to a nearby location within a short distance close enough from the oil palm plantations. Their stay in the oil palm land is not permanent for they must be prepared to relocate at any moment whenever the landowner asks them to leave. They are sometimes charged of making the oil palm area unclean and unsafe. Nonetheless, some groups of the Orang Rimba continue to pursue funeral ceremonies for a deceased family, just as their parents did; that is, they do not bury the corpse.

The *melangun* tradition, which used to last longer and be tied to death, has been performed with lesser intensity during the pandemic. It has also become linked to seeking sustainable livelihoods. However, when it comes to the practice of *melangun*, the Orang Rimba are diverse in its implementation. For the individuals who have settled permanently, the tradition is only carried out by a family member who is grieving the loss of the loved one. Those who reside near oil palm fields go through the *melangun* nearby their houses; it is not only because their living space is becoming increasingly limited but also because they have to restrain contacts with the outsiders during the COVID-19 pandemic.

The *melangun* tradition, i.e., fleeing their homes either to seek a new shelter, to dodge the death curse, or to discover a new hunting area is in fact favorable to reduce vulnerability to COVID-19. When people are leaving for a *melangun*, they are automatically avoiding crowds and contacts with the outsiders. Their access to social interaction is limited only to certain individuals who are mostly their relatives. When they are doing a *melangun*, they are actually engaged in what is, in its modern term, referred to as social distancing. In light of compliance with health protocols, nevertheless, their daily activities seems to be the same as they were before the pandemic. In day-to-day life, no one is wearing a face-mask due to both scarcity and inconvenience. They are not familiar with the idea of wearing a face-mask. They are living a relatively communal life isolated from the general societies and therefore wearing a face-mask is a practice totally alien to them.

In addition to the melangun, the Orang Rimba also holds a tradition of *besesandingon*, which in the context of COVID-19 means physical or social distancing. At the beginning of the pandemic, the Orang Rimba adapted by relocating to the forest and instituting a mechanism of distancing (*besesandingon*). This tradition has been passed down from generation to generation in an effort to prevent contagious diseases among the Orang Rimba. When an Orang Rimba is ill or has just come from outside the village, he or she will be segregated or quarantined and is not permitted to interact directly with the rest of the Orang Rimba. When we were visiting their locations, it appeared to us that *besesandingon*—which for the Orang Rimba means to maintain a safe distance from unknown outsiders—was not observed in a disciplined manner. According to one informant, however, some other groups of the Orang Rimba continued to rigidly adhere to *besesandingon* by refusing to meet outsiders who have an interest in them. On the other hand, when an outsider comes to them, the Orang Rimba likewise will keep a distance. In addition to maintaining a safe distance through *besesandingon*, they curtail their activities as part of their adaptation strategy.

As for the Nuaulu in Maluku, hunting traditions are considered physical exercises that can enhance the body's immunity. A student at the Faculty of Public Health, Airlangga University has conducted an interesting research on the Nuaulu's hunting practices under the title *Perilaku Berburu, Local Knowledge dan Keseimbangan Imunitas Masyarakat Suku Nuaulu di Daerah Endemi Malaria Pulau Seram* (Hunting Behavior, Local Knowledge and Immunity Balance of the Nuaulu in the Malaria Endemic Area of Seram Island). The study revealed that the hunting tradition does not cause malaria in the Nuaulu people, but rather brings a positive impact on health by activating and regulating food safety patterns. During hunting, the frequency with which the hunters consumed nutrient-dense foods was increasing, and their exposure to disease vectors and indigenous herbal remedies strengthened their immune systems (Marasabessy, 2019). If we put it into the context of the COVID-19 virus, and despite the need for deeper researches, it is not impossible that with such a lifestyle the Nuaulu people naturally have better immune systems than the urban communities who are susceptible to a variety of diseases due to a lack of physical activity.

In the context of population demography, the tradition of Tengger indigenous people in Ngadas Village is strongly related to women's reproductive health. This traditional ritual is carried out every three months even during the pandemic in accordance with health protocols involving medical experts. The tradition referred to here is *pethekan*, which continues to exist today. *Pethekan* is a tradition of prenatal tests for unmarried or widowed women of child-bearing age. The Tengger people care deeply about the sanctity of sex for which reason the *pethekan* ritual is observed. This is also directly tied to the popular belief that the presence of illegitimate pregnancies is marked by unusual nature signs and spread of disease (Abidin, 2018). Among the unfortunate consequences are: many residents suffer discomfort for no apparent cause; many of them, regardless of gender, feel like they are craving, and many children suddenly get ill. The unusual nature signs include a rooster crowing at midnight or a tiger is spotted entering the village. Therefore, the *pethekan* tradition is mandatory for all unmarried or widowed women of Ngadas Village and it takes place every three months at the house of Pak Legen (Abidin, 2018).

The term *pethekan* derives from the procedure performed for this ritual, which involves gently palpating the abdomen. "*Pethek*" itself is a Javanese word that means "being pressed (*ditekan*)."The tests are generally carried out every three months by a traditional birth attendant (*dukun bayi*), a midwife (*bidan*), and *legen* (an assistant to the *dukun bayi*). In the past, only traditional birth attendants were allowed to conduct the *pethekan* since they have the ability to check for pregnancy. However, modern scientific knowledge has been now included to ensure the accuracy of the test. Consequently, village midwives now take part in the *petheken* tradition.

In the context of women's reproductive health, the *pethekan* tradition has been assimilated with modern health science in an effort to pursue early detection of unwanted pregnancies as well as birth controls. This tradition is designed to prevent women, particularly the single or unmarried ones, in Ngadas Village from engaging in free sex behaviors truly harmful to their reproductive health. During the *petheken* procession, the traditional birth attendant and the village midwife examine each woman in one of the rooms at the Legen's house. The traditional birth attendant and then the village midwife will press a women's abdomen. Whenever pregnant symptoms are present, testing will be administered through scientifically-validated urine sample. When the examination is done, all the participants are not allowed to return home immediately; rather, they have to listen to the debrief delivered by traditional birth attendant and the midwife on reproductive health issues, such as the importance of protecting oneself from promiscuity, the risks of sex outside marriage and so forth. Thus, *pethekan* serves as a socio-cultural control against unwanted pregnancies and free sex activities for unmarried women of Ngadas Village.

If a woman is found to be pregnant outside of wedlock, the customary law stipulates that she must pay a fine of 50 sacks of cement. If the man and the women are both unmarried, each of them must pay a fine of 25 sacks of cement. However, the fine is increased to 100 sacks of cement if the man is a married person, and the fine should be paid within ten days by the latest. The cement will be utilized to support village facilities, such as repairing potholes, constructing neighborhood security posts and other public infrastructures. All the residents come out and mutually collaborate in these activities. Upon payment of the fee, the couple must get married as soon as possible.

The *pethekan* tradition held by the Tengger indigenous people in Ngadas Village is aimed to safeguard women's chastity and reproductive health as well as to spiritually protect the village against disease or pandemic. There is a popular belief among the Tengger people that an unwed pregnant woman, particularly if she goes for an abortion, is feared to bring plagues like the COVID-19 pandemic to their village. Thus, the Tengger people of Ngadas Village continue to perform the *pethekan* every three month during the COVID-19 pandemic.

5.2 Adaptation Strategies in the Socio-Economic-Cultural Domain During the Pandemic

a. Education

Education was one of the sectors directly impacted by the COVID-19 pandemic. Teachers and students are unable to interact directly, so face-to-face teaching and learning activities had to be modified. The national policy of the government mandates that all students should have their education through online at home (El Widad & Bakar, 2021; Winata et al., 2021). In 2020, the government, through Circular Letter of the Secretary General of the Ministry of Education and Culture No. 15 of 2020 concerning the Implementation of Learning from Home in the COVID-19 Emergency Period, issued an official command that schools should organize learning from home using online distance learning. Then, in 2021, a Joint Decree of the Minister of Education, Culture, Research and Technology No. 5/KB/2021, the Minister of Religion No. 1347 of 2021, the Minister of Health No. HK.01.08/Menkes/6678/2021, and the Minister of Home Affairs No. 443-5847 2021 concerning the Implementation of Learning during the COVID-19 pandemic was issued. Accordingly, this joint decree made some regions continue to engage in online education until 2021. This shift put forward additional requirements so hard to be fulfilled by the students with limited access to technology, such as the Orang Rimba, the Nuaulu, and the Marapu youngsters in Sumba, who live in remote areas without Internet connectivity (Sawitri, 2021; Talu et al., 2021; Tahir, 2021). The government policy that generalize online education for all students has undoubtedly posed new challenges. In the case of the Orang Rimba, limited access to technology eventually prevents them from attending school effectively. As a result, they frequently skip the class on purpose to follow their father hunting in the forest, which is more vital to their survival than attending school.

This circumstance necessitates adaptations distinct from those required for learning in urban areas where access to technology is more readily available. One strategy in the educational sphere that we observed was that the teachers are regularly visiting their students to teach. For instance, the teachers from Central Maluku traveled to the Nuaulu village of Nua Nea to educate their students. They gathered in one of the villager's house to engage in teaching and learning activities. Most of the elementary school pupils do not have cell phones or internet access, hence this strategy is deemed to be highly effective. The intermittent presence of the teacher was helpful to make sure the students, particularly those at elementary school level, are keeping with their studies. Meanwhile, the senior high school students can learn independently from home and utilize their cell phones to remain active in class.

b. Economy

The local government responded to the pandemic in accordance with the policies of the central government by imposing restrictions on physical activities and promoting healthy living behaviors, including the implementation of 3 M and even 5 M: always washing hands, wearing masks, maintaining distance, avoiding crowds, and refraining from eating together (Sutomo et al., 2021). As a consequence, several economic activities are not running as usual. In the case of Bali, for instance, the enactment of this policy has resulted in a decline in economic activity in addition to the closure of hotels and tourism facilities due to restrictions on the arrivals of domestic and foreign tourists. Most workers in the tourism industry suffered job losses (PHK), salary cuts due to reduced working hours, and temporary unemployment without a monthly paycheck.

During the COVID-19 outbreak, the Indonesian government has disbursed various aids to its citizens who are directly affected. It is envisaged that the aids worth a total of trillions of rupiah will lighten the burden on the people whose economies have been severely impacted by the virus. The government has distributed various types of aids during the pandemic, including basic foods, Social Cash Assistance (Rp600,000), Direct Cash Aid-Village Fund (Rp600.000), free electricity, pre-employment cards, employee salary subsidies, and Direct Cash Aid for micro and small businesses (Cantika, 2021; Retnaningsih, 2020; Titik & Nugroho, 2021; Yendra & Wetsi, 2021). The empowerment assistance program of the Ministry of Social Affairs for Remote Indigenous Communities (KAT) seems to be the most responsive and economically promising initiative for indigenous peoples. The Ministry of Social Affairs, through the Directorate General of Empowerment, has granted Cash Social Assistance (BST) to 2,500 Beneficiary Families (KPM) in 32 wards/villages of Suku Anak Dalam (SAD) (Ministry of Social Affairs, 2021). In 2021, the empowerment program targeted to empower 2,500 KAT households. The community has been using the government's aid as a part of their strategy to fulfill life's demands.

The local government of Negeri Nua Nea exemplifies how the government continues to take an active role in channeling programs to the community. Our interviews showed that when the pandemic is increasingly widespread and is slowing down the people's economy, the Negeri Nua Nea authorities began diverting around 30 percent of the village's budget for Direct Cash Assistance (BLT). It is worth mentioning that Negeri Nua Nea receives an annual Village Fund Allocation (ADD) of Rp800 million. During the pandemic, they allocated a portion of the ADD for Direct Cash Assistance to handle the COVID-19 crisis. The authorities dispersed health protocols-related items, such as face-masks and hand sanitizers, to the public. Financial aid worth of Rp300, 000 was also disbursed and distributed monthly to 52 families (State Apparatus, personal communication, 8 September 2021). The distribution of the Direct Cash Assistance was pursued with fairness and transparency. The residents who have never received government help through other programs (the PKH and BLT) was given priority to get COVID-19 crisis assistance. However, the decision to grant the BLT for COVID-19 also took into account the severity of the virus' impact on a family, especially considering that the majority of Nua Nea residents are categorized as poor. It is undeniable that the COVID-19 pandemic has lowered the income of people, particularly those who rely on the sale of plantation and agricultural goods.

The local government plays a crucial role in ensuring that government aid programs reach the community members (Lewis & Hendrawan, 2019; Pramono, 2019). The citizens' data collection is essential for the distribution of programs and aids during this pandemic. In addition to the government, NGOs serve as the government's collaborators in delivering empowerment support programs. One of them is Pundi Sumatra, which is pursuing to empower local communities, such as in Sarolangun District, with funding from the Ministry of Social Affairs. It has been currently running a program called The Second Year 2021 Social Empowerment

Program for Remote Indigenous Communities in Pematang Jumat, Limbur Tambesi Village, Bathin VIII Sub-District, Sarolangun District. The program is administered through the transfer of social assistance to the group's bank accounts. According to information provided by the NGO partner of Pundi Sumatra, one of the rather heavy indicators for the program is to measure progress on the basis of economic parameters.

Following up the PPKM policy, the government started delivering social aids to the community, although it could not reach everyone and was only for a short period of time. However, the government's policies were still limited to providing aids and did not include programs to strengthen the community's economic resilience in the face of difficult times. In addition to relying on the strategies being prepared by the government to overcome economic hardship during the pandemic, the local communities have launched a number of self-help initiatives event though in the face of the economic burden posed by the pandemic, not many alternatives were available. The optional natural resources were too limited to be maximized for alternate sources of income during the pandemic. However, the data at several research sites indicated that the pandemic has spawned other means of subsistence. In Sumba and Bali, for instance, it is evident that tourism-related activities have not been the main source of revenue and therefore could serve as additional sources of livelihoods.

The coping strategies adopted to address economic difficulties during the pandemic entail optimizing agricultural and plantation activities. During the pandemic, people has devoted more time to agriculture by laboring in gardens and cultivating edible and marketable products, such as tomatoes, corn, and vegetables. Finding it as the only possible opportunity to meet their financial demands, the community exerts more effort to develop their lands. For example, the fisherman of Wundi Village, Papua, have been optimizing copra processing for generating additional money for survival. As the fish sales are becoming sluggish due to a shortage of purchasers, the profits by selling copra to the collecting traders in Biak have provided them with an additional source of income.

The data finding from the other research sites confirmed that the local farmers utilize garden products to the greatest extent possible as part of their survival strategies. Garden commodities, such as sweet potatoes, corn, peanuts, and green beans, are not only sold but also kept to meet the family's dietary needs. When it came to vegetable commodities, the problem occurred when the pandemic hit and the policy of entry/exit access restriction was put in place in Biak; during the days, some farmers had no choice but to discard their vegetable products due to a lack of buyers.

As for the Orang Rimba in Jambi, our research findings showed that their coping strategies include establishing new sources of income through oil palm cultivation (for those who own land). When the prey animals are increasingly rare in the forest, they try their luck at planting oil palms and other money-making products.

The agricultural sector is most likely to absorb migrant workers returning to Bali. Some of them are working on land owned by their families, while others are cultivating someone else's land or becoming hired labor. Even though this agricultural activity does not immediately generate income, as the Perbekel of Banjar Asah

Gobleg said, the farming they undertake has been able to lift their family's food self-sufficiency. In the meanwhile, the village authorities seek to give mentoring for those who have lost or never had agricultural skills. This support program is not limited to providing temporary means of subsistence during the pandemic; it also aims to restore the former farmers' enthusiasm for farming and make the agricultural sector a priority in Asah Gobleg Banjar's economic development.

Like in Bali, the Tengger people of Ngadas employ their adaption strategy for preventing the spread of COVID-19 by disallowing tourists or visitors to come to Ngadas for tourism-related matters. When the area of Tengger was restricted to tourists during the PPKM, the tourism sector in the area was slowing down. In practice, they temporarily suspended many tourism-related activities. Consequently, they depended on their primary source of income as farmers for their survival tactics and adaptation during the pandemic. They returned to the agricultural sector as their primary livelihoods by planting potatoes in the fields.

This farmer-back-to-farmer activity is pursued not only by men. Instead of just staying at home, women are spending more time in the fields during the pandemic. Because the location between the fields are physically far apart, social distancing between the residents become inevitable. Furthermore, the people are relatively healthier due to easy access to naturally fresh air and clean water. By keeping the farming activities, they are able to sustain their economic base and generate sufficient cash to cover their needs while maintaining their health.

In addition, the pandemic has prompted social interactions in a number of regions with two or more distinct livelihoods, such as bartering between the farmers and the fisherman as a survival strategy in meeting food needs. For instance, fish collected by the fisherman is traded for tubers or vegetables harvested by the farmers, thereby enabling each party to fulfill their dietary needs. This pattern is prevalent among the Orang Asli Papua who still have relatives in the village or brothers of the same clan (*saudara semarga*) selling fish and agricultural items to the city. This situation particularly occurs in the urban areas where the residents returned to gardening activities due to their increased free time after the installation of WFH (work from home) as well as the belief that physical activity can strengthen their immunity against the COVID-19 virus.

The next coping strategy employed by the community is reducing food intake and/or cutting expenditures. During the pandemic, a decrease in income and lack of social aid have prompted the community to adjust by making the best use of available resources and reducing consumption. The food intake reduction is exemplified by, among many others, financial arrangement and/or the cutting of very costly protein consumption. One household would preferably eat vegetables, noodles, or eggs because they are more economical. In fact, they would usually reduce their eating frequency from three times to twice per day for which they felt satisfied enough. The enactment of the Emergency PPKM some time ago seemed to have caused many trade-dependent households to cut their daily expenditures. The data from Central Maluku indicated that reducing fish consumption becomes one of the simplest strategies to minimize family expenses (Resident of Rohua, Personal communication, 9 September 2021).

Another adaptation strategy to preserve the family economy is running economic activities as usual. The residents of Sumba, for instance, continued to produce woven goods and waiting for the tourism to resume that they can sell their products again. Despite all the limitations, fabric weaving activity remains active during the pandemic. Due to a decline in the amount of tourists visiting their village, the Marapu people sell their woven goods on the market. The woven products being sold are confined to woven materials typically used for ritual purposes.

c. Health

Community-wide vaccination is one technique for mitigating the adverse impacts of COVID-19 on health (Aminah & Susilo, 2021; Arifin & Anas, 2021; Toharudin et al., 2021). Nonetheless, this vaccination program continues to face many challenges in the field, such as a shortage of resources and public acceptance (Budiman & Chu, 2021; Faturohman et al., 2021; Harapan et al., 2020a; Harapan et al., 2020b). The role of the government in addressing COVID-19 among the Nuaulu people has not shown significant results or has not been maximized yet. In relation to the COVID-19 vaccination, the Central Maluku District Health Office has performed socialization in Negeri Nua Nea (Negeri Apparatus, Personal Communication, 8 September 2021). In fact, most people are still worried about the possible side effects of vaccination. Information has been widely circulated on Facebook claiming that vaccinations can cause death (Triwardani, 2021; Udhany & Sylvia, 2022). This has made the residents of Nua Nea reluctant to be vaccinated, especially when they feel in good health. Despite this, it is possible that this trend will change as the government put forward regulation on vaccination. For example, persons who intend to travel outside of the island have no choice but to provide proof of vaccination through the Peduli Lindungi application.

The apparatus and community leaders play a crucial role for the success of the vaccination program (Arief & Karlinah, 2019; Kamal et al., 2021). As the holders of governmental authorities, the village chief or administration, along with the staff, seek tirelessly to enforce health protocols. The village government also facilitates the vaccination program for its citizens, despite its imperfections. The findings in East Java indicated that the Village Government of Tengger Ngadas showed its commitment to the success of the vaccination program for all the residents. According to the most recent statistics, phase 1 vaccination has reached approximately 1,200 of the targeted 1,500 residents in Ngadas Village. The Village Chief, in his capacity as the head of the COVID-19 task force, claimed that in addition to the vaccination program, the Village Government has spent 8% of the village fund for the management and prevention of COVID-19, in accordance with the instruction from the central government. Various efforts have been made to promote vaccine take-up among the residents; for example, the village apparatus drove a car with a loudspeaker traveling around the community to inform the residents about the vaccination schedule.

The low level of community participation for vaccination is a quite complex issue for it is also related to the belief of indigenous peoples, not to mention the circulation of vaccine misinformation and hoaxes. Therefore, it is not surprising that most of indigenous peoples prefer to lean on traditional techniques, such as the use of traditional herbs, as their adaptation strategy against COVID-19 (Irwansyah, 2021; Subagyo & Harfiani et al., 2021). The findings in the Marapu village on Sumba indicated that indigenous people consume herbal remedies to treat coughs and lung problems. The people also express their concern about COVID-19 by pursuing to enhance their immune system. They have access to a variety of potions that they believe can block entry of viruses into their bodies. Many herbs they are familiar with are useful to heal coughs and even extreme colds. Among indigenous peoples, the COVID-19 symptoms, such as fever, cough, and headache, are still regarded as common ailments they are frequently afflicted with. According to the findings of studies on the forest-dwelling Orang Tugutil, herbs or forest potions have been used to treat all these types of illness. Similarly, in response to COVID-19 the Orang Rimba in Jambi continue to rely on traditional practices that they have faith in and inherited from their ancestors. They believe that sugar cane plants will shield their village from COVID-19 and other diseases.

One of the keys to containing the COVID-19 outbreak is minimizing interaction with outsiders and refraining from contacts with strangers (Saud et al., 2021). The alertness of Marapu people toward guests from outside the village represents at least their effort to protect their elderly people from direct contact with visitors. They will make a careful observation to ensure that the visitors do not carry the virus; provided that the proof has been established interaction will be permitted after several visits. The efforts to enforce health protocols are shown also in the office buildings and some of the major roads, despite the fact that at the time of data collection, only few COVID-19 cases were detected.

In addition, the implementation of health protocols is crucial the success of which will require collaborative efforts between the government, the community, and the individual (Fridayani & Soong, 2021; Maarif, 2021; Yodang et al., 2021). As the only region of the Nuaulu Tribe having a status of Administrative State (*Negeri Administratif*) in Central Maluku, it can be said that Nua Nea is more than ready to face the COVID-19 pandemic. This is shown by the presence of health protocol-supporting amenities, such as hand-washing stations, in public facilities. The Negeri apparatus placed hand-washing facilities with soap in front of the Negeri office or hall for it serves as a meeting place for Nua Nea's visitors. Furthermore, they also displayed banners advising the public to be more attentive against the spread of the COVID-19 virus. They put information regarding the COVID-19 symptoms and their preventative measures. The banner mentions nine preventative tips, including: (1) Drink warm liquids (preferably ginger coffee or tea); (2) Gargle every time with antiseptic and warm water; (3) Take a shower with soap every time you return from a trip or traveling; (4) Clean any metal surfaces. (5) Consume fruits and vegetables; (6) Animals do not transmit the coronavirus, it happens only between people; (7) Avoid the flu; (8) Soak up the sun from 9:00 to 10:00 in the morning; and (9) Always worship and pray to God.

The residents of Biak-Numfor considered COVID-19 as a common disease because it was not immediately noticeable to them. As a precautionary measure, they implemented health protocols, such as wearing face-masks when selling fish catch to Biak and garden vegetables at the market. Therefore, they continued to wear face-masks when they are in public spaces. The Papuan people are renowned for their robust physiques and high levels of immunity. Some healthy day-to-day exercises have become ingrained in the Papuan way of life. According to some informants, daily routine linked to the maintenance and improvement of the Papuan people's immunity included: (1) straightforward physical activities under the sun, both as farmers and fisherman; and (2) A nutritious diet of fresh sea fish and garden vegetables. Carbohydrates are provided by ingestion of rice and tubers interchangeably on a daily basis, while protein is derived from fish and pig; (3) More individuals are on foot when moving from one place to another; traditional remedies or herbs are still consumed to improve the body's immune system; and (4) No stress.

One important adaptation carried out by The Tenggers, particularly women, is making the best advantage of technology. Mutmainah, a village midwife at the Poncokusumo Community Health Center, said that COVID-19 had a significant impact on various parts of citizen health services, including Posyandu, Health Maintenance Support and Education (*Bina Sehat*), and basic vaccination, etc. Prior to the pandemic, all these activities were conducted normally and crowdedly. Since the COVID-19 pandemic, however, their interactions have been restricted. Consequently, the control over pregnant women by the midwives has been optimized through WhatsApp and other communication technologies.

5.3 The Synergy Between Indigenous Peoples and Local Government in the Face of the Pandemic

Synergy or collaboration that involves individual actors, communities, and state entities, is vital for coping with COVID-19. This cooperation at many levels becomes the key to successfully manage COVID-19 cases during the high waves of COVID-19 cases. In response to this pandemic, the strategies of individuals, communities, and government institutions in each location differ widely, seemingly becoming the strength that enables people to endure difficult circumstances. This section will elucidate how people, communities, and government institutions are working together to fight the pandemic. Layered synergies between individuals, government authorities, traditional and religious leaders have established a harmonious social interaction during the pandemic. Systematic recovery efforts are required at all levels, including the government, the private parties, the community, and non-governmental organizations. Protecting belief systems, values, and traditions must be the focus of institutional resilience enhancement (Lugo-Morin, 2021). Indigenous peoples in several countries, such as Bolivia, Mexico, and Peru, are using traditional medicine to prevent and treat the symptoms of the coronavirus among their communities. By maintaining traditional knowledge of healing plants and herbs and community self-care practices, they are also determined to revive their traditional medicine and self-care treatments. Although the efficacy of these practices in preventing COVID-19 infection and treating the disease is still unknown, the use of these traditional remedies has enabled indigenous peoples to take necessary measures to combat the pandemic within their communities (OHCHR, 2020).

a. Individual Actors

At the personal level, the synergy between communities took place in numerous ways. Even though it should be admitted that in the context of indigenous peoples, individual concerns are not the focal point because social proximity remains the top priority. In the case of the Orang Rimba, individual actors such as *jenang* serve as the intermediaries between the Orang Rimba and outsiders, including the government and non-governmental organizations. The Orang Rimba has been always vulnerable during this pandemic. Individually, they adjust by avoiding crowds, engaging in forest-related activities, and relying on traditional medicine, among other things. Exposure to information related to COVID-19 that they received from their fellow villagers tends also to contain false information. Tracing and vaccination rates are still relatively low among the Orang Rimba. In the context of the Orang Rimba in Jambi, the role of *jenang* as a liaison and a non-governmental organization (NGO) at the local level is crucial for the successful management of the pandemic, both in terms of the provision of social aid and the vaccination program. As for the Tengger people, synergy is carried out through technology. The mothers are using WhatsApp and other communication technologies to gain access to health services such as Posyandu, Health Maintenance Support and Education (Bina Sehat), and basic vaccination. This condition helps them avoid the crowd during formal occasions. Meanwhile, individuals and households among the Merapu people of NTT are trying to survive the pandemic on their own. Various efforts are carried out at the household level, such as optimizing activities in agriculture and plantations, reducing food intake, striving to boost the body's immunity by the use of traditional herbs, restricting interactions and producing woven fabric. Relations between individual actors are forged with a common goal to survive difficult situations and, therefore, are utilized in practice to increase health and sustain economic demands.

b. Community

Community is a crucial force in combating the COVID-19 pandemic. At the community level, many patterns and strategies are employed to organize strengths in response to the pandemic, beginning with the management of food stockpiles, medicine, and other aspects, as well as the development and administration of the various support networks available (Rippon et al., 2020). At the community level, synergies have been implemented in several regions to combat the pandemic. In the Tengger people of Ngadas, at the local level the village chiefs collaborate with the religious leaders to address the challenging circumstances caused by the pandemic. For example, the combination of cultural-religious and formal approaches channeled by the village government at the local level has successfully facilitated the enforcement of health protocols. Despite its imperfections, the village authorities have been doing their best to make vaccinations easily accessible to the residents. The local government has also allotted a budget for the vaccination program. In addition, the shaman as a holder of customary authority also plays a crucial role, for example, by leading a particular ceremonial procession known as "*Nyangoni*" or "providing supplies or *sangu*" to protect the community against COVID-19. The synergy between the village leaders or chiefs and religious leaders (Hindus, Buddhists, Muslims, Christians) is exemplified by conducting a joint prayer for protection from God.

In Bali, the traditional village chiefs play a significant role in combating the pandemic. The religious leaders, traditional village headman (*bendesa adat*), and health professionals (*balia usada*), as Sugi Lanus (a Balinese philologist) said, were among the first to respond to the pandemic by issuing a joint decision, known as *pararem*, on how to handle it in the areas of traditional villages. The *pararem* put forward instructions on restricted ceremonies, medical treatments, quarantine, burial, and cleansing rituals. As is the case in Munduk Village, which is part of the Catur Desa Adat Dalam Tamblingan, the *bendesa* plays a key role in dealing with COVID-19 by, for example, serving as a member of the mutual cooperation task force whose responsibility is to promote health protocols and rituals of ward off misfortune (*tolak bala*).

The Merapu people of NTT adheres strictly to their customs (*adat*). They performed collaboratively the ritual of ward off misfortune (*tolak bala*) with the hope that the pandemic will end as soon as possible. Indigenous groups, such as those residing in Kampung Tarung, also carried out traditional rites. In October and November, the Wula Pollu traditional ceremony was held with the participation of all society elements and the presence of various parties. The purpose of the Wula Pollu ceremony is to invoke God's gift and blessing of salvation. The community's synergistic collaboration was instrumental for the successful performance of this traditional ceremony.

To prevent the spread of COVID-19 in Central Maluku, the Nuaulu indigenous people of Rohua worked together to organize the Usi Rosa ceremony in October 2020. This traditional procession was aimed to atone for misdeeds and was attended by all adult residents of Rohua who still stick to their indigenous beliefs. This mass activity involved more than one hundred Rohua locals. Even though not all Nua Nea's residents complied with the health protocols, the important role of traditional elders in their implementation should not be underestimated. Despite the fact that not a single person in the Negeri was willing to wear a face-mask, the Father King (*Bapa Raja*) recommended his people to wear a face-mask when traveling to Masohi City for trade or other essential purposes.

As for the Orang Tugutil, no synergy was visible at the community level because the COVID-19 case had no effect on their socio-demographic situations. On this aspect, it is important to develop family- and community-based alternative health systems in order to strengthen the Orang Tugutil's capacity in coping with the COVID-19 pandemic and other infectious diseases in the future. In the case of Biak, there existed social exchanges at the community level, which consisted of commodity barters between farmers and fishermen as a survival strategy to meet their food demands. This traditional act of trading goods take place among the Orang Asli Papua (OAP) with close familial links regardless of their different occupations as farmers and fishermen. For instance, seafood captured by fishermen is exchanged for tubers or vegetables so that both parties can meet their food needs. The OAP maintain kinship bonds with their relatives in the village or with their brothers of the same clan selling fish and agricultural goods to the city.

c. Government Institutions

The role of government institutions is the primary driving force behind the management of the pandemic. The government has well-defined structures and has already outlined pandemic management protocols to be implemented down at the local level (Ministry of Health, 2021). In addition, the government has also put Remote Indigenous Communities (KAT) into the scheme of the Social Safety Net (JPS) program by providing Cash Social Assistance (BST) and basic foods (Ministry of Social Affairs, 2020). Nonetheless, there are evidence that demonstrate the government's shortcomings in managing the pandemic. In the case of the Orang Rimba in Jambi, for instance, the population registration data of the Orang Rimba has not been adequate, which to some extent hindered the identification of Orang Rimba for the COVID-19 aid handling programs. The accuracy of population statistics has a significant impact on the provision of government aid, as the distribution of various government supports requires a proof of residence identity.

In Ngadas, East Java, the village chief and the staff, who serve as the holder of authority at the village level, represent the role of government institutions. The village government has been vigorously enforcing health protocols and facilitating vaccination program though not yet optimal. The community reported that they do not receive any kind of COVID-19-related social aid. The reason is very fundamental in that the government's support would go to those who need it most.

In Bali Province, the COVID-19 task force becomes an extended hand of the government in coping with the pandemic at the village level. A strong collaborative effort between community groups at the village level is a powerful weapon in combating the pandemic. The *Bendesa* (Traditional Village Chief; Klian Adat) and *Perbekel* (the Official Village Chief), along with other community groups, have developed a number of projects to mitigate the effects of the pandemic by maximizing the village's available resources. In this role, the *Perbekel* acts as an extension of the government, whose main responsibility is to implement government initiatives, such as health protocols and cash and non-cash aid distribution. In Asah Goblek Banjar, the Perbekel has been proactive in registering the village community groups who had come back after voluntarily going away from home (*merantau*).

As in other regions, the government has also implemented the PPKM policy in NTT in order to cut down the virus transmission. The government shut down tourist infrastructure and facilities, as well as banned tourist visits. The provincial and district governments has also offered food assistance and household needs during the period of activity restrictions. In addition, the social supports were given to the beneficiaries.

In Central Maluku, the active participation of the Nuaulu indigenous people in managing COVID-19 has not yet reached a significant level. The government has been attempting to socialize the vaccine despite unproven results. The District Health Office of Central Maluku has also conducted dissemination in Nua Nea. As of September 8, 2021, only four individuals were willing to receive the first vaccine dose (Negeri Apparatus, Personal communication, September 8, 2021). The government has been unsuccessful in persuading those who remain concerned about vaccination side effects. In addition to vaccination program, the local administration has been seeking to enforce health procedures and social aid for low-income individuals. When the virus hit and affected the population's economy, the Negeri apparatus in Nua Nea began allocating around 30 percent of the village's budget for direct cash aid (BLT). The Negeri apparatus of Nua Nea has been also looking to accelerate the administration process of Indonesia Health Card (KIS) for the residents (Resident of Nua Nea, Personal Communication, September 8, 2021).

In North Maluku, the government has not done maximum efforts in delivering social assistance funds. When it came to giving COVID-19 related assistance programs to the Orang Tugutil, particularly those living in the forests, the problem arose as they refused to accept aid directly from the hands of strangers. The donations from the local government being offered by the government officials, for instance, had to be stored in front of them before being received. The local governments all the way down to the village level collaborate to promote the habits of wearing a face-mask, washing hands, maintaining physical distance, avoiding crowd, and restricting mobility. Nevertheless, the Orang Tugutil did not entirely comply with these practices. In Biak, Papua, a variety of aid has been disbursed to help relieve the burden on the shoulders of the people, ranging from food assistance, cash social aid (Rp600,000), BLT-village funds (Rp600,000), free electricity, pre-employment cards, wage subsidy schemes, to BLT for micro and small businesses.

References

Abidin, M. Z. (2018). Tradisi petekan dan upaya mencegah kehamilan di luar nikah pada masyarakat suku tengger. *Journal de Jure, 10*(2), 89–97. https://doi.org/10.18860/j-fsh.v10i2.6725

Aminah, S., & Susilo, S. R. T. (2021). State capacity in implementing the COVID-19 vaccination program in Indonesia. *Advances in Social Science, Education and Humanities Research, 560*, 67–72. https://doi.org/10.2991/assehr.k.210615.014

Arief, N. N., & Karlinah, S. (2019). The role of Ulama (Islamic religious leaders) in countering anti-vaccination rhetoric in Indonesia. *Journal of Asian Pacific Communication*. https://doi.org/10.1075/japc.00038.ari

Arifin, B., & Anas, T. (2021). Lessons learned from COVID-19 vaccination in Indonesia: Experiences, challenges, and opportunities. *Human Vaccines & Immunotherapeutics*, 1–9. https://doi.org/10.1080/21645515.2021.1975450

Budiman, D., & Chu, C. (2021). A SWOT analysis of Indonesia's COVID-19 pandemic response strategy. *International Journal of Advanced Health Science and Technology, 1*(2), 50–52. https://doi.org/10.35882/ijahst.v1i2.3

Cantika, D. A., Yulandari, F. H., Arriski, F., & Al A, H. F. (2021). Bantuan sosial COVID-19 dalam perspektif ekologi administrasi. *Jurnal Dialektika: Jurnal Ilmu Sosial, 19*(2), 12–22. https://doi.org/10.63309/dialektika.v19i2.3

Daulay, Z. (2012). Tatakelola perlindungan pengetahuan obat tradisional: Keberpihakan kepada kepentingan rakyat banyak. *Masalah-Masalah Hukum, 41*(2), 288–297.https://doi.org/10.14710/mmh.41.2.2012.288-297

El Widad, Z., & Bakar, M. Y. A. (2021). Wajah baru pendidikan Indonesia di masa pandemi dan analisis problematika kebijakan pendidikan di tengah pandemi. *Jurnal Mappesona, 4*(1), 1–12. https://www.jurnal.iain-bone.ac.id/index.php/mappesona/article/view/1768

Faturohman, T., Kengsiswoyo, G. A. N., Harapan, H., Zailani, S., Rahadi, R. A., & Arief, N. N. (2021). Factors influencing COVID-19 vaccine acceptance in Indonesia: An adoption of technology acceptance model. *F1000Research, 10,* 1–23. 10.12688%2Ff1000research.53506.2.

Fridayani, H. D., & Soong, J. J. (2021). The emergent role of local government on COVID-19 outbreak In Indonesia: A new state-society perspective. *Journal of Governance, 6*(1), 23–45. https://doi.org/10.31506/jog.v6i1.10287

Harapan, H., Wagner, A. L., Yufika, A., Winardi, W., Anwar, S., Gan, A. K., Setiawan, A. M., Rajamoorthy, Y., Sofyan, H., Vo, T. H., Hadisoemarto, P. F., Müller, R., Groneberg, D. A., & Mudatsir, M. (2020a). Willingness-to-pay for a COVID-19 vaccine and its associated determinants in Indonesia. *Human vaccines & immunotherapeutics, 16*(12), 3074–3080. https://doi.org/10.1080/21645515.2020.1819741

Harapan, H., Wagner, A. L., Yufika, A., Winardi, W., Anwar, S., Gan, A. K., Setiawan, A. M., Rajamoorthy, Y., Sofyan, H., & Mudatsir, M. (2020b). Acceptance of a COVID-19 vaccine in Southeast Asia: A cross-sectional study in Indonesia. *Frontiers in Public Health, 8,* 381. https://doi.org/10.3389/fpubh.2020.00381

Harfiani, E., Puspita, R., & Ramadhani, I. (2021). Characteristics of Indonesian society in utilizing herbs for Covid prevention during the COVID-19 pandemic. In *SIOP Conference Series: Earth and Environmental Science* (Vol. 913). https://doi.org/10.1088/1755-1315/913/1/012104

Iwuoha, V. C., & Aniche, E. T. (2020). COVID-19 lockdown and physical distancing policies are elitist: Towards an indigenous (Afro-centred) approach to containing the pandemic in sub-urban slums in Nigeria. *Local Environment, 25*(8), 631–640. https://doi.org/10.1080/13549839.2020.1801618

Kamal, A., Rubin, J., & Rogers, B. (2021). Using behavioral science to develop public health messages for racial and ethnic minority communities during COVID-19. 1–18. https://doi.org/10.1038/s41562-020-0884-z

Kotala, S., & Firdhausi, N. F. (2019). Keanekaragaman tumbuhan berkhasiat obat pada suku Noaulu di Pulau Seram, Maluku. *Biotropic: The Journal of Tropical Biology, 3*(1), 49–55. https://doi.org/10.29080/biotropic.2019.3.1.49-55

Kristiyanto, E. N. (2017). Kedudukan kearifan lokal dan peranan masyarakat dalam penataan ruang di daerah. *Rechts Vinding, 6*(2), 151–169. https://doi.org/10.33331/rechtsvinding.v6i2.172

Kristiawan, J., Prasetijo, A., & Sutiningsih, D. (2021). & nbsp; Ketahanan pangan KKeluarga Orang Rimba Selatan Taman Nasional Bukit Dua Belas Jambi: Studi mikroetnografi keluarga Njalo dalam menghadapi pandemik. *Jantro 23*(1). https://doi.org/10.25077/jantro.v23.n1.p83-92.2021

Lewis, B. D., & Hendrawan, A. (2019). The impact of majority coalitions on local government spending, service delivery, and corruption in Indonesia. *European Journal of Political Economy, 58,* 178–191. https://doi.org/10.1016/j.ejpoleco.2018.11.002

Lugo-Morin, D. R. (2021). Global mapping of Indigenous resilience facing the challenge of the COVID-19 pandemic. *Challenges, 12*(1), 15. https://doi.org/10.3390/challe12010015

Maarif, S. (2021). Re-establishing human-nature relations: Responses of indigenous people of Indonesia to COVID-19. *Interdisciplinary Journal for Religion and Transformation in Contemporary Society, 7*(2), 447–472. https://doi.org/10.30965/23642807-bja10023

Marasabessy, N. B. (2019). Perilaku Berburu, Local Knowledge dan Keseimbangan Imunitas (TNF Alpha & IL-10) pada Masyarakat Adat Suku Nuaulu di Daerah Endemis Malaria Pulau Seram. [Doctoral Dissertation, Universitas Dipenogoro]. http://repository.unair.ac.id/id/eprint/86113

Ministry of Health. (2021). *Protokol tatalaksana COVID-19 di Indonesia* (edisi ke-2). Kementerian Kesehatan. https://covid19.go.id/artikel/2021/02/08/protokol-tatalaksana-covid-19-di-indonesia

Ministry of Social Affairs. (2020). Bantuan sosial tunai: Penyambung asa di tengah rimba. https://kemensos.go.id/bantuan-sosial-tunai-penyambung-asa-di-tengah-rimba

Ministry of Social Affairs. (2021). *Tahun 2021, Kemensos targetkan berdayakan 2.500 KK Warga KAT.* https://kemensos.go.id/tahun-2021-kemensos-tergetkan-berdayakan-2500-kk-warga-kat

Muchammad, E. B., Kurniawati E., Rozakiyah, D. S. (2021). Resiliensi Pelaku Wisata Masyarakat Desa Ngadas dalam Menghadapi Pandemi COVID-19. *Sosietas 11*(2), 123–134. https://doi.org/10.17509/sosietas.v11i2.41609

Nasruddin. (2010). Kearifan lokal dalam *pappaseng* Bugis. *Sawerigading,* Vol. 16, No. 2, Agustus 2010.

OHCHR. (2020). COVID-19 and Indigenous Peoples' Rights. https://www.ohchr.org/Documents/Issues/IPeoples/OHCHRGuidance_COVID19_IndigenouspeoplesRights.pdf

Pramono, D. R. (2019). Peran pendampingan dalam pelaksanaan Bansos Non Tunai Program Keluarga Harapan (PKH). *Journal of Social and Political Science, 1*(2), 69–75. https://jurnal.unej.ac.id/index.php/jsps/article/view/13618

Prasetijo, A. (2017). Livelihood transformations of the Orang Rimba as tacit resistance in the context of deforestation. *Endogami: Jurnal Ilmiah Kajian Antropologi, 1*(1), 1. https://doi.org/10.14710/endogami.1.1.1-13

Radhia, H. A. (2021). Adat Istiadat dan Kerukunan Umat Beragama Masyarakat Tengger. In C. Saputra & R. Suriaputra. *Imajinasi Nusantara: Budaya Lokal dan Pengetahuan Tradisional dalam Masyarakat Indonesia Kontemporer*. 62–78. PSIK, Kemenko PMK RI, & FriedrichEbert-Stiftung.

Retnaningsih, H. (2020). Bantuan Sosial bagi Pekerja di tengah Pandemi Covid-19: Sebuah analisis terhadap kebijakan sosial pemerintah. *Aspirasi: Jurnal Masalah-Masalah Sosial, 11*, 215–27. https://doi.org/10.22212/aspirasi.v11i2.1756

Rippon, S., Bagnall, A. M., Gamsu, M., South, J., Trigwell, J., Southby, K., Warwick-Booth, L., Coan, S., & Woodward, J. (2020). Towards transformative resilience: Community, neighbourhood and system responses during the COVID-19 pandemic. *Cities & Health.* https://doi.org/10.1080/23748834.2020.1788321

Rumilah, S., Nafisah, K. S., Arizamroni, M., Hikam, S. A., & Damayanti, S. A. (2020). Kearifan lokal masyarakat Jawa dalam menghadapi pandemi. *SULUK: Jurnal Bahasa, Sastra, Dan Budaya, 2*(2), 119–129.

Saud, M., Ashfaq, A., Abbas, A., Ariadi, S., & Mahmood, Q. K. (2021). Social support through religion and psychological well-being: COVID-19 and coping strategies in Indonesia. *Journal of Religion and Health, 60*(5), 3309–3325. https://doi.org/10.1007/s10943-021-01327-1

Sawitri, S. (2021). COVID-19: Tingkat stres belajar anak-anak di daerah terpencil. *Al-Madrasah: Jurnal Pendidikan Madrasah Ibtidaiyah, 5*(2), 101–124. https://doi.org/10.35931/am.v5i2.542

Setyowati, M. F. (2003). Hubungan keterikatan masyarakat kubu dengan sumberdaya tumbuh-tumbuhan di Cagar Biosfer Bukit Duabelas Jambi. *Biodiversitas Volume 4, Nomor 1,* 47–54. http://citeseerx.ist.psu.edu/viewdoc/download?doi=10.1.1.675.799&rep=rep1&type=pdf#page=51

Steinebach, S. (2012). *Der Regenwald ist unser Haus-die Orang Rimba auf Sumatra zwischen Autonomie und Fremdbestimmung.* Universitätsverlag Göttingen. https://library.oapen.org/bitstream/handle/20.500.12657/32551/610299.pdf?sequence=1

Subagyo, F. A. K. D., & Irwansyah, I. (2021). Cognitive dissonance in health-seeking behavior of people in Indonesia to prevent COVID-19. *SALAM: Jurnal Sosial dan Budaya Syar-i, 8*(1), 251–266. https://doi.org/10.15408/sjsbs.v8i1.18692

Sutomo, S., Sagala, S., Sutomo, B., Liem, W., & Al Hamid, H. (2021). Strengthening the strategic and operational response for reducing COVID-19 transmission in Indonesia. *Kesmas: Jurnal Kesehatan Masyarakat Nasional (National Public Health Journal).* https://doi.org/10.21109/kesmas.v0i0.5104

Tahir, S. Z. B. (2021, March). Designing English teaching model at the remote area schools of Maluku in COVID-19 pandemic situation. In *Proceedings of the 11th Annual International Conference on Industrial Engineering and Operations Management.* Universitas Iqra Buru https://repository.ejournal-uniqbu.ac.id/publications/345465/designing-english-teaching-model-at-the-remote-area-schools-of-maluku-in-covid-1#cite

Talu, M. M., Kristanto, W. H., & Santhalia, P. W. (2021). Efektivitas pembelajaran Fisika daring di era pandemi COVID-19 pada sekolah yang kesulitan akses internet (Studi Kasus Sekolah di Kabupaten Sumba Barat). *Jurnal Penelitian Pembelajaran Fisika, 12*(2), 196–202.

The Committee for the Coordination of Statistical Activities. (2020). *How COVID-19 is changing the world: a statistical perspective.* UNSTATS. https://unstats.un.org/unsd/ccsa/documents/covid19-report-ccsa.pdf

Titik, C. S., & Nugroho, R. Y. Y. (2021). Respon awal petani, nelayan, dan usaha mikro, terhadap bantuan COVID-19. *e-Journal Ekonomi Bisnis dan Akuntansi, 8*(1), 8–19. https://doi.org/10.19184/ejeba.v8i1.21374

Toharudin, T., Pontoh, R. S., Caraka, R. E., Zahroh, S., Kendogo, P., Sijabat, N., Sari, M. D. P., Gio, P. U., Basyuni, M., & Pardamean, B. (2021). National vaccination and local intervention impacts on covid-19 cases. *Sustainability, 13*(15), 8282. https://doi.org/10.3390/su13158282

Triwardani, R. (2021). Indonesian officials and media fight vaccine hesitancy, misinformation. *Asian Politics & Policy, 13*(4), 635–639. https://doi.org/10.1111/aspp.12608

Tumenggung Tarib. (2012). Kesaksian Tumenggung Tarib "Orang Rimbo" Provinsi Jambi disampaikan pada sidang perkara nomor 35/PUU-X/2012, perihal pengujian Undang-Undang Nomor 41 Tahun 1999 tentang Kehutanan terhadap Undang-Undang Dasar Negara Republik Indonesia Tahun 1945 di Mahkamah Konstitusi Republik Indonesia [Court testimony]. Mahkamah Konstitusi Republik Indonesia.

Udhany, D., & Sylvia, S. (2022). New media literature: An effort to combat the COVID-19 Vaccine Hoax in Indonesia. *Budapest International Research and Critics Institute (BIRCI-Journal), 5*(1), 2363–2373. https://doi.org/10.33258/birci.v5i1.3838

United Nations. (2020). COVID-19 and Indigenous peoples. https://www.un.org/development/desa/indigenouspeoples/covid-19.html

Winata, K. A., Zaqiah, Q. Y., Supiana, S., & Helmawati, H. (2021). Kebijakan pendidikan di masa pandemi. *Ad-Man-Pend: Jurnal Administrasi Manajemen Pendidikan, 4*(1), 1–6. https://doi.org/10.32502/amp.v4i1.3338

Yendra, M., & Wetsi, W. P. M. (2021). Dampak Bantuan Langsung Tunai (BLT) dana desa COVID-19 terhadap perekonomian masyarakat. *Jurnal Ilmiah Ekotrans & Erudisi, 1*(2), 14–22. https://doi.org/10.31933/jiee.v1i2.409

Yodang, Y., Kiik, S. M., Fauji, A., Hamka, H., Pratiwi, R. M., Nuridah, N., & Fitrina, Y. (2021). Knowledge, attitudes, and practices of Indonesian residents regarding covid-19: A national cross-sectional survey. *International Journal of Public Health Science, 10*(2), 418–427. https://doi.org/10.11591/ijphs.v10i2.20722

Chapter 6
Conclusion: Lessons Learned from the COVID-19 Pandemic for a Better Future

Sari Seftiani and Cahyo Pamungkas

Abstract This chapter is a conclusion that offers the lesson learned from the COVID-19 pandemic through a socio-demographic perspective. Socio-demographic conditions and the COVID-19 pandemic have a two-way relationship. On the one hand, the socio-demographic characteristics of a given country or region can increase its vulnerability to COVID-19. On the other hand, the COVID-19 pandemic has directly and indirectly significant impacts on socio-demographic circumstances. Given that this pandemic is not the first nor will it be the last, it is crucial to socio-demographically understand COVID-19 and how to handle it. The recent pandemic should serve as a big lesson to prepare well in the face of any similar or worse event that may occur in the future. Moreover, it is essential to see the COVID-19 pandemic not only as a health concern but also in relation to other aspects. This book, which comes from the findings of collaborative research conducted by the BPS and the BRIN in 2021, focuses on indigenous communities as an object of research. Indigenous people are categorized as one of the vulnerable groups during the current COVID-19 pandemic. The narrative that has been constructed thus far pertaining to the vulnerability of indigenous peoples is that they are currently dealing with many challenges, such as marginalization, poverty, lack of access to facilities, loss of land rights, etc. However, the fact shows that indigenous peoples with local wisdom are arguably more resilient to the COVID-19 pandemic than other community groups. Reflecting on the research's findings in this book, we call attention to some aspects that have been neglected by the government in dealing with the crisis. The governmental regime ideologically driven by developmentalism and the neoliberal economy tends to become "authoritarian" and unwilling to listen to civil society by nature. This is evident from its pandemic-related responses and policies that came a bit "late" during the early phase of the COVID-19 outbreak. A lesson learned from our research findings is that addressing

S. Seftiani (✉)
Research Center for Population, National Research and Innovation Agency (BRIN), Jakarta, Indonesia
e-mail: sari.seftiani@brin.go.id

C. Pamungkas
Research Center for Area Studies, National Research and Innovation Agency (BRIN), Jakarta, Indonesia

C. Pamungkas et al. (eds.), *The Impact of the Pandemic on Indigenous People in Indonesia*, Quality of Life in Asia 20, https://doi.org/10.1007/978-981-96-4222-9_6

the COVID-19 pandemic will require the participation of multiple parties—i.e., the central government, regional governments, scientists/academics, commercial actors, and the community—in order to develop resilient systems for crisis. Collaboration and partnership are essential given that the pandemic and its effects are complex, and, therefore, dealing with them will need the participation of all stakeholders. In this sense, the government's technocratic and bureaucratic approaches to the pandemic do not solve the problem. Rather, optimization in handling the impacts of the pandemic and in building future resilience should entail community participation through a variety of community asset-based social innovations at the local level.

Keywords Indigenous people · COVID-19 pandemic · Socio-demographic · Vulnerability · Resilience · Government

Socio-demographic conditions and the COVID-19 pandemic have a two-way relationship. On the one hand, the socio-demographic characteristics of a given country or region can increase its vulnerability to COVID-19. On the other hand, the COVID-19 pandemic has directly and indirectly significant impacts on socio-demographic circumstances. Given that this pandemic is not the first nor will it be the last, it is crucial to socio-demographically understand COVID-19 and how to handle it. The recent pandemic should serve us a big lesson to prepare well in the face of any similar or worse event that may occur in the future. Moreover, it is essential to see the COVID-19 pandemic not only as a health concern, but also in relation to other aspects.

This book, which comes from the findings of collaborative researches conducted by the BPS and the BRIN in 2021, focuses on indigenous communities as an object of scrutiny. Indigenous people are categorized as one of the vulnerable groups during the current COVID-19 pandemic. The narrative that has been constructed thus far pertaining to the vulnerability of indigenous peoples is that they are currently dealing with many challenges, such as marginalization, poverty, lack of access to facilities, loss of land rights, etc. However, the fact shows that indigenous peoples with local wisdom are arguably more resilient to the COVID-19 pandemic than other community groups.

The indigenous peoples in this book are, broadly speaking, refer to groups of individuals who share the same cultural traits (cultural staff); they also belong to shared beliefs and senses of belonging to a group that is distinct from others. Not only do indigenous peoples share the same culture or social system, but some of them were also founded on the belief that they come from the same lineage or ancestors. One of them is referred to as the Marapu indigenous people on the island of Sumba. Most of the traditions that have been passed down for generations by the people of Sumba are believed to have originated from the Marapu beliefs, which are, for the most part, kept alive today. This conception follows Weber (1978) in defining ethnic groups as described in Chapter 2. Disagreement over the concept of indigenous peoples or communities is not the focal point of discussion in this book. In this regard, indigenous peoples in Indonesia are so diverse that there is no single definition for what and how they are.

As described in Chapter 2, the perspective employed in this book rests on approaches to cultural traits. One of them is Koentjaraningrat's (2004) description of ethnic groups, which refer to collectivities whose members share common cultural traits such as language, belief systems, rituals, and other cultural symbols. Obviously, the dimension of these cultural traits coexists with the social one, which is preservation of social borders through contact or interaction, rather than isolated living areas. These ethnic groups, let's say the Marapu people, realize that they are a distinct group, and another group, let's say Kupang people, recognize this differences within an inter-ethnic interaction. Therefore, cultural and social dimensions are the main basis for this book in defining indigenous peoples as ethnic groups.

6.1 Understanding the COVID-19 Pandemic Through Socio-Demographic Aspects

6.1.1 Indigenous Populations' Vulnerability to the COVID-19 Pandemic

The primary focus of this book is to present a socio-demographic analysis of the COVID-19 pandemic. As indicated previously, socio-demographic factors can be used as indicators to determine the level to which a region or a population is susceptible to the COVID-19 pandemic. In addition, demographic data is also helpful to predict from the beginning the spread of COVID-19 cases, on the basis of which policies on measures to mitigate the pandemic's effects can be properly made. This demographic data applies not only to indigenous populations but also to society as a whole. Unfortunately, according to the findings of the research jointly conducted by the BPS and BRIN, the availability of demographic data on indigenous peoples in Indonesia, particularly in terms of COVID-19 exposure, is still very limited. This should be an important note that the availability of complete and reliable data is an instrumental aspect in coping with the pandemic. The lack of an agreed-upon definition of indigenous peoples by government institutions and civil society organizations makes the condition even worse.

Age structure, gender, population mobility and density, livelihoods, and cultural or ritual activities stand out as five socio-demographic characteristics that increase the vulnerability of an area or a population to the COVID-19 pandemic. Seen from the age structure, the elderly population, i.e., those aged 60 years and older, is at a greater risk of death from COVID-19 than other age groups. Despite the fact that the vast numbers of positive COVID-19 cases are found among those in productive age, the mortality rate among the elderly is significantly higher. Age is crucial in understanding the disparity in COVID-19-related mortality risk. Moreover, age is an indicator for the progressive accumulation of permanent damage over the course of a lifetime, and is hence strongly related with chronic illness and disability (Nepomuceno et al., 2020). Indigenous populations with a high proportion of elderly people are more susceptible to death when exposed to COVID-19 due to their increased mortality risk. The indigenous peoples of Tengger, Bali, and Marapu have a relatively high number of elderly people.

Gender can serve as an indicator of susceptibility to COVID-19. Positive COVID-19 cases between men and women are not significantly different. However, fatalities are higher in male patients. In line with the research findings done by Balbo et al. (2020a, 2020b), the mortality rate from COVID-19 tends to be disproportionately greater in men and those with comorbidities. A study in Indonesia confirmed this, arguing that a higher proportion of active smokers among men may be one of the variables increasing the severity of the COVID-19-related disease (Susilo et al., 2020).

Population mobility is the most influential demographic indicator on a region's susceptibility to the COVID-19 pandemic. In an area with high population mobility, the risks of COVID-19 transmission is significantly greater. According to a research (BPS-BRIN), a considerable number of COVID-19 cases is found in areas with extensive population mobility. In addition, an increase in COVID-19 cases frequently occurs along with the loosening of people's movement, particularly with regard to restrictions on travel outside the region and overseas. In Indonesia, COVID-19 cases are known to have surged after the celebrations of Eid Al-fitr, Christmas, and New Year's Eve.

Meanwhile, settlement patterns associated to population density also affects susceptibility to the spread of COVID-19. It is quite often that indigenous peoples adopts to a compact and closely built pattern of housing. For example, in the Nuaulu people of Central Maluku and the Marapu of Sumba Island, East Nusa Tenggara Province, their settlement patterns are relatively clustered and near together in one village. Because they are living in one village, they feel no need to implement tight health protocols. A research by BPS-BRIN revealed the fact that one village experienced symptoms of illness similar to COVID-19, particularly loss of smell.

Regarding economic activities, indigenous peoples' livelihoods also determine both their susceptibility to COVID-19 infection and the severity of its effects. During the pandemic, agriculture and plantations have provided a rather stable source of income for sustaining daily needs. Moreover, the agricultural sector of indigenous peoples is typically subsistence-based and some are small-scale economic business. In addition, the residents who rely on agriculture for a living tend to be sedentary and therefore they have a lower risk of COVID-19 exposure. Similar to those who depend on tourism-led livelihood, they rarely meet people outside their village.

Meanwhile, traditional ceremonial activities or cultural traditions that are held in a public space and are not only attended by members of the community, but also by people from outside the community are one of the factors that can make indigenous peoples more vulnerable to the spread of COVID-19 cases. Cultural or customary activities usually draw a large crowd and therefore heighten vulnerability, especially in tourist destinations. There is a widely held concern that such activities will open doors for the spread of COVID-19 unless they are staged in accordance with health protocols. In addition, the coming of visitors from outside the region to watch the events can magnify the level of vulnerability to the spread of COVID-19.

6.1.2 *The Impacts of the COVID-19 Pandemic on Indigenous Populations*

The COVID-19 pandemic, has significantly impacted and severely disrupted people's lives. The COVID-19 pandemic has put challenges on many facets of life, including socio-economic and demographic conditions, both directly and indirectly. The study conducted by the BPS-BRIN demonstrated that population mobility and migration are demographic aspects most affected by the pandemic. The imposed policies of restricting population mobility have directly or indirectly systemic effects on other areas of life. This regulation has exerted a considerable pressure on livelihoods, particularly for those who rely on the tourism sector. The decline in tourist visits resulted in a significant decrease in revenue.

The COVID-19 pandemic has an indirect impact on births (fertility). Although the impact on births (fertility), which is also a socio-demographic aspect, is not as big as what happens to population mobility and migration, there are signs of a possible increase in the number of births in the following years. The number of births tended to be steady; however, the qualitative study showed an interesting finding that there has been a decline in the usage of contraceptives (KB) in some research sites, including Bali and Central Maluku. One of the reasons is that people were reluctant to visit health facilities due to a fear of being exposed to or tested positive for COVID-19. The statistical data analysis from the 2020 Population Census showed, for instance, a rise in the Child Women Ratio (CWR) in Biak-Numfor in 2020 as compared to 2010, which also indicated an increasing birth rate in this region. This can also mean that the indigenous Papuans made an effort to avoid the depopulation of the Orang Asli Papua already happening in the coastal regions of Papua Land. The initial conclusion that can be inferred is that although there has not been a statistically significant rise in the birth rate during the pandemic, there is a tendency for changes in reproductive health-related behaviors that may have an impact on future birth rates.

The most obvious direct impact of demographic aspect is mortality. Since the COVID-19 cases were first detected in Indonesia in March 2020, this virus has caused a significant number of deaths. Except for indigenous peoples in Bali, the death toll among indigenous peoples was low in general. Bali is one of Indonesia's provinces with a high fatality rate. Indirectly and directly, the pandemic had a significant impact on Bali's indigenous population. However, the lack of ethnicity-based data could be one of the reasons why the exact numbers of death rates among indigenous peoples are hardly possible to achieve. Whereas, many members of indigenous peoples refused to get COVID-19 tests despite having the symptoms; they also avoided health facilities in the fear of contracting the coronavirus during the pandemic. In fact, the BPS-BRIN study (2021) found in the research site that people living in one village with close-knit communities exhibited symptoms identical to those of COVID-19, such as loss of smell.

Meanwhile, the government's various policies and programs enacted in reaction to the COVID-19 pandemic affect indirectly the implementation of social, economic, and cultural activities among indigenous populations. In general, there is little change in terms of cultural activities or customs. Numerous traditional activities are still taking place but participation in some of them is restricted. In the context of the COVID-19 pandemic, cultural activities are not necessarily prohibited, but it is only that they may potentially cause large crowds that can facilitate the transmission of the disease. A traditionally well-established perception that the failure to conduct ritual will bring bad luck is a factor that contributed to the continued performance of those activities. In addition, the traditional rites being held is believed to have gathered only participants from a given village and its nearby surroundings and are, therefore, safe from the coronavirus.

The economic impact is deeply experienced by all levels of society, particularly indigenous peoples who depend on tourism-led livelihoods. A significant drop in income and loss of employment are the two dominant indirect impacts of COVID-19. Various measures restricting population movement have reduced the number of migrants in the tourism sector. Indigenous peoples who work in the tourism sector experience a greater economic losses than their fellows in the agricultural and plantation spheres. Even though they suffer a decrease in income due to the weakening power and values of their agricultural and plantation sales, they are still able to carry out their routine agricultural activities and to utilize their farm or garden products for daily consumption in order to survive the pandemic.

6.2 How Do Indigenous Peoples Respond and Adapt to the COVID-19 Pandemic?

Many consider indigenous peoples to be one of the most vulnerable groups, even prior to the outbreak of the COVID-19 pandemic. Chapter 3 showed that indigenous populations are susceptible to the COVID-19 pandemic, as seen from their age distribution and economic activities. The effects of COVID-19 on indigenous populations are also quite diverse and impacted by numerous factors. In response to this, strategies for surviving the COVID-19 pandemic have been developed. In the context of the COVID-19 pandemic, indigenous peoples with local knowledge are typically more resilient to withstand the pandemic than the broader communities.

Responses and adaption strategies are shaped by perceptions on which information, knowledge, experience, and culture have an influence. The ways indigenous peoples perceive and understand the COVID-19 pandemic are socially constructed and shaped by a variety of related social situations, such as daily and past life experiences, the number of cases, and technology and social media-driven information or news circulating about the coronavirus. It can be argued that numerous indigenous peoples have a relatively low perception of the threats posed by COVID-19. This is due in part to the experience of illnesses with almost identical symptoms to COVID-19 and a variety of other previous disasters that, in their views, had a greater impact than the COVID-19 pandemic. However, it should also be noted that this relatively low perception is influenced in part by lower rates of COVID-19 cases in their region. The majority of indigenous peoples in this study tend to be "reluctant" to wear a face-mask for various reasons related to their knowledge. Face-masks are only worn when entering the city, leaving the village, or stepping into an office. The widely circulated COVID-19-related narratives among the indigenous peoples in the research sites include, among others, that COVID-19 only occurs in urban areas like Jakarta, that migrants from outside the area are the most heavily affected, that COVID-19 is a seasonal flu disease, and that patients are "being deliberately diagnosed with COVID-19" ("*dikovidkan*") by the hospitals. All these popular opinions exert an impact on the manner in which indigenous peoples respond to the COVID-19 pandemic, particularly in terms of their health-related behavior for prevention and treatment. As an example, in the case of Bali, many COVID-19 deaths are attributable to people avoiding in-hospital tests; accordingly, COVID-19 positive individuals with comorbidities are most likely to suffer more severe health problems due to lack of intensive medical check-up.

Another response to the COVID-19 pandemic involves maintaining a safe distance and avoiding crowds. It is difficult for indigenous peoples to keep physical distance from people and stay away from crowded areas, especially when attending or participating in cultural rituals or activities. Despite instructions on restricting activities, indigenous peoples continue to engage in crowds-gathering cultural and traditional events, making it impossible to maintain physical distance. The perception that their region belongs to the green zone of COVID-19 cases and that the activity is carried out by the villagers who have known each other is one of the reasons behind the continued activities.

Intriguingly, despite all these low-level perception of COVID-19, indigenous peoples are strategically pursuing to avoid the coronavirus by relying on their existing local knowledge, particularly in health behavior for prevention and treatment. In almost all research locations, the belief in traditional herbs allegedly considered effective in curing diseases with symptoms similar to COVID-19 sustains the health behavior of indigenous peoples in facing the pandemic. In addition to healing, it is believed that their traditional herbs can maintain the body's immune system throughout the pandemic. In fact, some indigenous peoples being encountered in this study are confident that the herbs had successfully prevented them from COVID-19 exposure.

At the community level, indigenous peoples have undertaken numerous responses and adaptation measures, such as the ritual of ward off misfortune (*tolak bala*), joint prayers, and social supports for the victims and afflicted communities. The ritual of *tolak bala* seeks to prevent disasters and other awful things. Some indigenous peoples, such as the Nuaulu Tribe, believe that natural calamities are caused by the errors of individuals and groups. This indigenous people collectively constructed a myth that a disaster is meant to be a "warning" or "reprimand" for mankind due to their numerous transgressions. By performing the ritual of *tolak bala*, which also contains prayers of sin confession, it is believed that a bigger calamity has been escaped.

In regard with adaptation on the economic aspect, a decrease in income as an indirect effect of COVID-19 has led to numerous survival strategies, such as job diversification, product marketing on social media, fabric production for the needs of traditional ceremonies (the Marapu), and simplified consumption of daily foods. Indigenous peoples who rely on the tourism sector, such as the Bali people and the Marapu believers in Sumba Island, have experienced a significant decline in income. Whereas, indigenous peoples that depend on the plantation sector do not suffer a large decrease in revenue, since they are still able to meet their daily needs through garden produce and forest hunting.

In addition, the COVID-19 pandemic has become a momentum showing that tourism-led livelihood is a highly vulnerable sector. Many indigenous peoples who first spent more time making a living from this sector are now returning to their agricultural land or plantations. Although some tourism-related businesses, such as the production of souvenirs and fabric, are still maintained, plantation or agricultural land has become the primary source of income or daily necessities during the pandemic.

6.3 Preparing for the Next Pandemic: What Have We Learned so Far?

The COVID-19 pandemic, which first broke out in December 2019 in Wuhan, China, and entered Indonesia in March 2020, has made it clearer that this country and many others across the world are not sufficiently prepared to deal with the disaster caused by the abrupt outbreak of the pandemic. The high rates of COVID-19-related fatalities and the inadequacy of health care facilities to accommodate COVID-19 patients are the clear evidence. Besides Indonesia, countries such as the United States, the United Kingdom, and Russia also reported significant fatalities due to COVID-19. Therefore, it is imperative to build preparedness and contingency strategies for calamities, including health disasters. The COVID-19 pandemic is not the first catastrophe in the world, nor will it likely be the last.

Based on the research findings presented in the preceding chapters, this book concluded that a study of socio-demographic conditions is pivotal for the foundation of policy- and decision-making during a pandemic-driven crisis. The government should take socio-demographic factors into account when making policies in times of crisis. There is a need for a deeper understanding of other issues than health. As previously explained, age structure can be a factor by which COVID-19 pandemic vulnerability is measured. On the other side, the pandemic also contributed to demographic shifts, such as an increase in mortality and a decrease in population mobility and migration. Moreover, welcoming an increasing older population amid the crisis also presents significant challenges. In this scenario, Indonesia tends to be reactive and lacks the initiative to develop resilient of human resources. This situation cannot be separated from Indonesia's peripheral position and its dependence on the structure of the global political economy.

Furthermore, the COVID-19 pandemic has shown that the elderly population is the most vulnerable group because they accounted for a majority of COVID-19 deaths. Although the rate of exposure to COVID-19 is higher among the productive-age people, due in part to their increased mobility, the death rate is higher among the elderly. Nearly half of COVID-19 cases among elderly people in Indonesia resulted in death. In the context of the indigenous peoples being studied, the 2020 Population Census data showed that the proportion of aged people, such as the Tengger indigenous people of East Java, the Marapu people of Sumba Island in NTT, and the indigenous peoples in Bali Province, has surpassed 10 percent. According to the World Health Organization (WHO), the proportion of the elderly above 10 percent is considered high. Even if there is a disparity in the proportion of aged persons among indigenous peoples, the descriptions of the three indigenous groups indicate a demographic shift toward an aging population. In addition, building and improving resilience in the face of calamities, particularly a health disaster, should be a top priority given that Indonesia is now entering a period of aging population (Seftiani, 2022). The question is to what extent infrastructure and health services improve rapidly and prepare for future pandemics amid aging population.

This qualitative study found that the high death rate among the elderly, such as in Bali, is due to the fact that, despite having comorbidities, they tended to avoid hospitals or other health facilities when exposed to COVID-19. Therefore, COVID-19 did not directly cause the mortality, but because the elderly had comorbidities and received no intensive treatment from medical workers, because of which their health conditions deteriorated and resulted in deaths. In addition, there is also reluctance to visit hospitals while experiencing COVID-19 symptoms due to the fear of being hospitalized under health protocols and far away from the family. An interesting finding came up in regard with the indigenous peoples of the Nuaulu and Marapu tribes. Some of the older adults being encountered claimed to still feel well and able to manage COVID-19. They tended to believe in the efficacy of traditional herbs that they have consumed so far to boost endurance and treat ailments, particularly those caused by COVID-19. The local knowledge of traditional herbs gives them some more confidence in their ability to avoid the coronavirus. Such a conviction on the local knowledge regarding medicinal herbs does not exclusively belong to the elderly people but also to nearly all indigenous peoples. In this aspect, it is necessary to understand health behavior in order to explain how indigenous peoples have developed distinct survival strategies against the COVID-19 pandemic.

Furthermore, the government has not paid much attention to the existence of indigenous peoples despite attempts of recognition were made through the 2012 Decree of the Constitutional Court. The Remote Indigenous Community Program seems to be nothing more than a "project" designed to entice the deep forest-dwelling members of indigenous groups to move out and live permanently in the settlements located on the forest's borders or on the side of the main roads. A limited amount of basic public amenities have been granted to the indigenous peoples living in the settlements after being "guided" ("*dibina*") by the Government. However, this guidance policy does not go any further to recognize and protect their fundamental rights, such land and its natural habitats.

However, in times of crisis caused by the pandemic, it turned out that indigenous peoples or communities provide many lessons learned to the public societies whom the modern world referred to as "civilized societies." For instance, several indigenous peoples have in fact engaged in traditional "physical distancing" in their daily lives. In the past, many of them preferred to settle in the deep forests or upstream areas of the rivers to avoid mandatory forced labor imposed by local authorities and Dutch colonialism. Another example is that before the pandemic, these communities were "relatively" dependent on the modern economy growing in urban areas, particularly for access to industrial products and money economies. During the pandemic, however, the vast majority of them have come to realize that agriculture (hunting or gathering), shifted cultivation, subsistence farming, and small-scale farming are the last bastion to protect economic, social, and cultural life. The COVID-19 pandemic has become a turning point for the resurrection of the previously abandoned agricultural sector. During the pandemic, agriculture has proven to be a steadier livelihood. Thus, the government should also respond to the adaptation strategy of indigenous peoples in times of crisis while pushing traditional agricultural economy to grow and advance as the primary repertoire in the story of socio-economic development.

Finally, reflecting on the research's findings in this book, we call attention to some aspects that have been neglected by the government in dealing with crisis. The governmental regime ideologically driven by developmentalism and neoliberal economy tends to become "authoritarian" and unwilling to listen to civil society by nature. This is evident from its pandemic-related responses and policies that came a bit "late" during the early phase of the COVID-19 outbreak. A lesson learned from our research findings is that addressing the COVID-19 pandemic will require the participation of multiple parties—i.e., the central government, regional governments, scientists/academics, commercial actors, and the community—in order to develop resilient systems for crisis. Collaboration and partnership are essential given that the pandemic and its effects are complex and, therefore, dealing with them will need the participation of all stakeholders. In this sense, the government's technocratic and bureaucratic approaches to the pandemic does not solve the problem. Rather, optimization in handling the impacts of the pandemic and in building future resilience should entail community participation through a variety of community asset-based social innovations at the local level.

References

Balbo, N., Billari, F., & Melegaro, A. (2020a). The strength of family ties and COVID-19. Contexts, American Sociological Association.

Balbo, N., Kashnitsky, I., Melegaro, A., Meslé, F., Mills, M. C., de Valk, H., & de Vilhena, D. V. (2020b, Mei). Demography and the coronavirus pandemic. https://www.population-europe.eu/files/documents/pb25_COVID-19.pdf

Koentjaraningrat. (2004). Kebudayaan, Mentalitet dan Pembangunan. Gramedia.

Nepomuceno, M. R., Acosta, E., Alburez-Gutierrez, D., Aburto, J. M., Gagnon, A., & Turra, C. M. (2020). Besides population age structure, health and other demographic factors can contribute to understanding the COVID-19 burden. *Proceedings of the National Academy of Sciences, 117*(25), 13881–13883

Susilo, A., Rumende, C. M., Pitoyo, C. W., Santoso, W. D., Yulianti, M., Herikurniawan, H., ... & Yunihastuti, E. (2020). Coronavirus disease 2019: Tinjauan literatur terkini. *Jurnal penyakit dalam Indonesia, 7*(1).

Seftiani, S. (2022). Learning from Pandemic COVID-19 Toward Ageing Societies in Indonesia: Building Resilience with Adaptive Social Protection. *Masyarakat Indonesia, 48*(2), 237–247. https://doi.org/10.14203/jmi.v48i2.1245

Weber, M. (1978). Economy and Society, ed. G. Roth and C. Wittich, University of California Press.

The manufacturer's authorised representative in the EU is Springer Nature Customer Service Centre GmbH, Europaplatz 3, 69115 Heidelberg, Germany. If you have any concerns regarding our products, please contact ProductSafety@springernature.com

Printed and bound by CPI Group (UK) Ltd, Croydon, CR0 4YY
30/09/2026
02225309-0003